W9-AVI-331

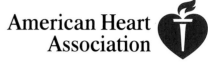

American Heart
Association

Learn and Live®

Pediatric Emergency Assessment, Recognition, and Stabilization
PROVIDER MANUAL

Editors

Mark Ralston, MD
Oversight Editor
Mary Fran Hazinski, RN, MSN
Senior Science Editor
Stephen M. Schexnayder, MD
Arno L. Zaritsky, MD
Monica E. Kleinman, MD

Special Contributors

Brenda Drummonds, *PEARS Writer*
Frank Doto, MS, *Senior Oversight Editor*
Louis Gonzales, NREMT-P, *Senior Oversight Editor*

American Academy of Pediatrics Reviewers

Susan Fuchs, MD
Wendy Simon, MA

Subcommittee on Pediatric Resuscitation 2007-2008

Monica E. Kleinman, MD, Chair
Arno L. Zaritsky, MD, Immediate Past
    Chair, 2006-2007
Marc D. Berg, MD
Aaron Donoghue, MD, MSCE
Diana G. Fendya, RN, MSN
Bradley S. Marino, MD, MPP, MSCE
Timothy R. Myers, RRT-NPS
Lester Proctor, MD
Faiqa A. Qureshi, MD
Elise W. van der Jagt, MD, MPH
Dianne L. Atkins, MD
Jeffrey Perlman, MD
Wendy Simon, MA
Sharon E. Mace, MD
Michael Sartorelli, MD
Michael G. Tunik, MD
Allan R. de Caen, MD
Michelle Terrell, APRN
Mark A. Terry, EMT-P
Stephen M. Schexnayder, MD
Melinda Fiedor Hamilton, MD, MSc
Reylon Meeks, RN, MS, MSN, EMT, PhD
Alson S. Inaba, MD

ISBN 978-0-87493-535-6

Contents

Part 6:
Management of Shock

Part 7:
Cardiac Arrest

Part 8:
Resuscitation Team Concept

Appendix

Student CD Contents

Contents

Preface

The Pediatric Emergency Assessment, Recognition, and Stabilization (PEARS) Course is a new offering that seeks to better meet the educational needs of AHA program participants. While Basic Life Support (BLS) is essential for all healthcare providers, not every provider who encounters children needs the full Pediatric Advanced Life Support (PALS) Course. Specifically, many providers must recognize a child with a potentially life-threatening condition and enlist the help of more advanced providers. Because the recognition of such children is paramount to improving outcomes, this course focuses on pediatric assessment and recognition skills with lesser emphasis on management.

The course is the product of several years' work with third-year medical students at the University of Arkansas College of Medicine. We are particularly grateful to Henry C. Farrar, MD, and Richard T. Fiser, MD, for their dedicated work in the development and execution of a prototype that formed the seminal base for this course. We acknowledge the support of the Betty Ann Lowe Distinguished Chair in Pediatric Education that fostered the initial course development. This course has been further evaluated and modified to better meet the needs of multiple audiences, including prehospital healthcare providers, in-hospital providers outside of critical care areas, outpatient clinic staff, and school-based providers.

Many dedicated volunteers and staff in the Emergency Cardiovascular Care Programs of the American Heart Association have invested thousands of hours in the development of this course. We hope that these efforts improve the care for critically ill and injured children by better meeting the educational needs of those who care for these most vulnerable patients.

Stephen M. Schexnayder, MD
Immediate Past Chair
Pediatric Resuscitation Subcommittee

Part 1

General Concepts

Introduction

Welcome to the **P**ediatric **E**mergency **A**ssessment **R**ecognition and **S**tabilization (PEARS) Provider Course. It is our hope that as a result of taking this course you will be able to

- recognize a seriously ill or injured child using the general and primary assessments
- understand and apply the "assess-categorize-decide-act" approach
- demonstrate effective CPR
- stabilize a seriously ill or injured child
- practice effective team interaction

The Purpose of This Manual

This manual provides background information to help you recognize a seriously ill or injured child (or infant) and determine if the child has a respiratory problem, a circulatory problem, or both.

The earlier you detect respiratory distress, respiratory failure, or shock and start appropriate actions, the better chance the child has for a good outcome.

The goal is to stop progression toward heart and lung (cardiopulmonary) failure and cardiac arrest. Once cardiac arrest occurs, outcome is generally poor. Only 5% to 12% of children who experience cardiac arrest in the out-of-hospital setting survive to hospital discharge. The outcome is somewhat better for children who experience cardiac arrest in the in-hospital setting: about 27% survive to hospital discharge.[1]

> *Your timely intervention may save the life of a child. If you recognize respiratory distress or shock and intervene quickly, you may prevent progression to cardiac arrest.*

Figure. Pathway to pediatric cardiac arrest.

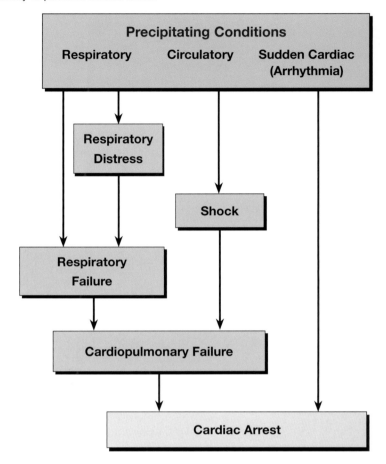

Note that respiratory conditions may progress to respiratory failure with or without signs of respiratory distress. Respiratory distress occurs when the child fails to maintain an open airway or adequate respiratory effort and is typically associated with altered level of consciousness. Sudden cardiac arrest in children is less common than in adults and typically results from arrhythmias, such as ventricular fibrillation or ventricular tachycardia.

Student CD

The student CD contains supplementary material to help you prepare to successfully participate in the PEARS Provider Course.

Topic	Description	How to Use
Resuscitation team concept	Discusses the role of the team leader and team members: explains the 8 elements of effective team dynamics	Read before the course so that you are prepared to participate as a team member in 8 case simulations during the course
Respiratory resources	Resources and procedures for managing respiratory distress or failure, eg, oxygen delivery systems, bag-mask ventilation	Review as necessary to prepare for the skills stations and case simulations; you must demonstrate competency in these skills according to your scope of practice
Circulatory resources	Resources and procedures for managing circulatory emergencies, eg, operation of a monitor/defibrillator in AED mode	
Intraosseous (IO) access	Procedure for performing IO access	Can be used as an optional learning station during the course
Chain of Survival	AHA Pediatric Chain of Survival illustrating a sequence of critical actions to reduce the risk of cardiac arrest in children	Read to understand the shared responsibility of the community at large, caregivers, and healthcare professionals in saving children's lives
Safety and prevention	Scene assessment for out-of-hospital providers	Read to increase your knowledge of this topic

Detailed and Advanced Concepts

This symbol is used to indicate more detailed or advanced concepts. Much of this content was developed by the American Heart Association Subcommittee on Pediatric Resuscitation. The information is based on years of experience and research in the field of pediatric advanced life support.

Part 2

Pediatric Assessment

Approach to Pediatric Assessment

Introduction

Use the "assess-categorize-decide-act' approach when caring for a child who is seriously ill or injured:

- *assess* the child using the general and primary assessment
- *categorize* the child's condition by type and severity
- *decide* what needs to be done
- *act* to provide appropriate treatment

You should repeat the "assess-categorize-decide-act" approach after any intervention or change in the child's condition.

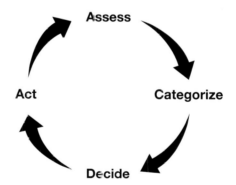

> *If at any point you identify a life-threatening problem, immediately start lifesaving actions and get help.*

Learning Objectives

After completing this part you should be able to

- discuss the "assess-categorize-decide-act" approach
- explain the purpose and components of the general assessment (pediatric assessment triangle)
- summarize the ABCDE components of the primary assessment
- explain the implications of clinical findings during the general and primary assessments
- evaluate respiratory and/or circulatory problems using the ABCDE model
- decide if a child has a life-threatening condition

Assess

Assess the child using a systematic approach. The pediatric assessment has 4 parts:

- General assessment[2]
- Primary assessment
- Secondary assessment*
- Tertiary assessment*

Below is a brief description of these clinical assessments. The *PEARS Provider Manual* discusses the general and primary assessments in detail. PALS providers usually perform the secondary and tertiary assessments. These terms suggest a sequential assessment. In reality several parts of each assessment are completed at the same time. You should adjust your assessment approach based on the child's clinical condition and history.

*Secondary and tertiary assessments will not be covered in the PEARS Course. You can find more information about these assessments in the *PALS Provider Manual*.

Clinical Assessment	Description
General assessment (pediatric assessment triangle)	The general assessment is a quick impression of what you see and hear regarding the child's • overall appearance • work of breathing • circulation Look and listen to assess the child within the first seconds of encounter. The pediatric assessment triangle represents this assessment.
Primary assessment	The primary assessment, or "ABCDE assessment," is a hands-on evaluation of the child. Each letter represents one part of the assessment: **A**—Airway **B**—Breathing **C**—Circulation **D**—Disability **E**—Exposure As part of this assessment you will check the child's • vital signs (including blood pressure and oxygen saturation by pulse oximetry) • blood glucose level
Secondary assessment	The secondary assessment is • a focused medical history using the SAMPLE mnemonic • a thorough head-to-toe physical examination
Tertiary assessment	The tertiary assessment consists of laboratory, radiographic, and other tests. These tests help establish the child's physiologic condition and diagnosis.

Note: In an out-of-hospital setting, always assess the scene to make sure it is safe before you assess the child.

 See "Scene Assessment for Out-of-Hospital Providers" on the student CD.

Categorize

Based on your assessment, try to categorize the child's clinical condition by type and severity. In this book we discuss categorization of respiratory and circulatory problems by severity first and then by type. In reality you will categorize both the severity and type of the child's condition at the same time.

Problem	Type	Severity
Respiratory	• Upper airway obstruction • Lower airway obstruction • Lung tissue disease • Disordered control of breathing	• Respiratory distress • Respiratory failure
Circulatory	• Hypovolemic shock • Distributive/septic shock • Cardiogenic shock* • Obstructive shock*	• Compensated shock • Hypotensive shock

The PEARS Provider Course does not cover recognition or treatment of cardiogenic and obstructive shock.

The clinical condition may include both respiratory and circulatory problems. As a seriously ill or injured child gets worse, one category of problems may lead to others. For example, a child with shock may develop respiratory distress. A child in cardiopulmonary failure has both respiratory failure and shock (usually hypotensive). This condition immediately precedes cardiac arrest.

> Note that in the initial phase of your evaluation, you may be uncertain about the type or severity of problems or both. It is important to reconsider your initial impressions as you continue or repeat your assessment.

Categorization of the child's condition is important because it helps you decide the best course of action.

Decide

Decide what to do based on your assessment and initial categorization of the child's clinical condition. Base these decisions on your scope of practice and the actions you are permitted to perform.

Act

Act to stabilize the child. Do what is appropriate for the type and severity of the clinical condition.

Actions for PEARS providers may include

- getting help by activating a medical emergency or rapid response team
- starting CPR
- obtaining an AED, code cart, or monitor/defibrillator
- placing the child on a monitor and a pulse oximeter
- positioning the child
- giving oxygen
- providing nebulizer therapy or using an epinephrine autoinjector

The best action may be to get help. You should provide the emergency support that the child needs until help arrives. Be prepared to assist as a member of the team after more advanced providers take over the child's care.

Transition of Care

It is important to continue providing lifesaving actions until other rescuers take over the care of the child. If you are providing CPR, don't stop abruptly when help arrives! Continue CPR if indicated. Give a summary of what happened and what you and others have done.

Reassess

The cyclic process of "assess-categorize-decide-act" is a continuous one. Reassess the child as you provide initial stabilization. For example, if you give oxygen, then reassess the child. Is breathing a little easier? Are color, oxygen saturation, and level of consciousness improving? After you give a fluid bolus to a child in hypovolemic shock, does circulation improve? Is another bolus needed?

> *Remember that the best approach is continuously to assess, categorize, decide, and act.*

General Assessment

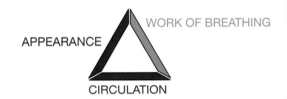

APPEARANCE   WORK OF BREATHING

CIRCULATION

Overview

The general assessment is the first and most basic assessment that you perform in the first seconds of patient encounter. This assessment is based on what you see and hear. The pediatric assessment triangle (PAT) represents these 3 components:

- appearance
- work of breathing
- circulation

The purpose of this assessment is to quickly identify a life-threatening condition. Assess the child's appearance, work of breathing, and circulation at the same time.

If the condition is ...	Then the next action is to ...
life threatening	• start life support actions • get help
not life threatening	continue with the next part of the assessment

Refer to the "Assess-Categorize-Decide-Act" (ACDA) Worksheet as you learn about assessment. This worksheet is located in the Appendix. During the course you will use it as an aid to recall the components of the pediatric assessment during discussions of video cases.

Appearance

Carefully observe the child during the first seconds of encounter. Gather as much information as you can about the adequacy of oxygenation, ventilation, and circulation. When assessing the child's appearance, note the level of consciousness. Is it normal or abnormal? Is the child less responsive or more irritable? Is the child unusually irritable?

If the child is crying or upset, it can be difficult to accurately evaluate her level of consciousness and interactivity. Try to keep the child as calm as possible during your assessment of appearance. Let her remain with her parent or caregiver if practical. Use distractions such as toys.

The "Tickles" (TICLS) mnemonic can help you recall characteristics of a child's overall appearance. Evaluate each characteristic. *Is it normal or abnormal?*

Characteristic	Normal	Abnormal
Tone (Muscle tone, movement)	Good tone; moves arms and legs well	Floppy or rigid; not moving
Interactiveness (Response to environment)	Responsive to parents or stimuli such as lights, keys, or toys	Decreased response
Consolability (Ability to be comforted)	Comforted	Not comforted in caretaker's arms; appears agitated or in pain
Look/Gaze	Opens eyes spontaneously; follows movement	Eyes closed; opens eyes only to verbal or painful stimuli; vacant stare
Speech/Cry	Normal speech or cry	Abnormal or absent

Work of Breathing

During the first few seconds, assess the child's work of breathing *without a stethoscope*. Observe the respiratory rate. Look for signs of increased or decreased respiratory effort. Listen for sounds of abnormal breathing. One primary purpose of this component is to decide if the child is in respiratory distress, respiratory failure, or respiratory arrest. Assess the following signs. *Is the work of breathing normal or abnormal?*

Sign	Normal	Abnormal
Respiratory effort*	• Breathing is regular with little apparent effort • Expiration occurs passively	• Nasal flaring • Chest retractions or abdominal muscle use • Increased, decreased, or absent respiratory effort
Airway sounds*	Breathing is without audible respiratory sounds	Noisy breathing—wheezing, grunting, stridor

*See the detailed discussion of respiratory effort and airway sounds in the section on primary assessment.

Circulation

During the first few seconds, assess signs of circulation. You can often find out important information about the child's circulatory status. When the amount of blood pumped by the heart (cardiac output) is too low, the body reduces circulation to nonessential areas such as the skin and mucous membranes. This is an attempt to preserve blood supply to the brain and heart. Thus, skin color and overall skin appearance provide important clues to help answer these questions:

- Is cardiac output adequate?
- Is blood flow to the brain and heart adequate?

Pallor (paleness), mottling (an irregular skin color), and cyanosis (bluish color) in the arms and legs may be signs of inadequate cardiac output and circulation. Central cyanosis may be present if the child is unable to adequately oxygenate the blood.

Observe the exposed parts of the child, such as the face, arms, and legs. Inspection of the skin may reveal bruising that suggests injury or trauma. You may also see evidence of bleeding within the skin, called petechiae or purpura.

Inspect the skin and mucous membranes. *Are they normal or abnormal?*

Sign	Normal	Abnormal
Skin color*	Appears normal	• Pallor • Mottling • Cyanosis
Hemorrhage	No obvious bleeding	• Obvious significant bleeding • Bleeding within the skin (eg, petechiae or purpura)

*See the discussion of skin color in the section on primary assessment.

Determine if the Child's Condition Is Life Threatening

Based on the information you gather during the general assessment, determine if the child's condition is

- life threatening
- not life threatening

If the child's condition is life threatening, start lifesaving actions and get help. (See "Life-Threatening Conditions" later in this part.) If the condition is not life threatening, you often will have an initial impression of whether the child has a respiratory or circulatory problem. Continue the primary assessment to better determine the clinical category and severity of the child's condition.

 Sometimes a child's appearance might seem normal, but the child could have a potentially life-threatening problem. An example is a child who has ingested a toxin. He may not yet be showing the effects of the toxin. Another example is an injured child with internal bleeding. The child's body may initially maintain blood flow to vital organs by increasing heart rate and narrowing blood vessels.[2]

These conditions show why it is important to repeat your assessment. Remember that the child's clinical condition will often change over time.

Primary Assessment

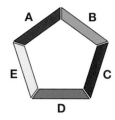

Overview

The primary assessment uses an ABCDE approach to assess

- **A**irway
- **B**reathing
- **C**irculation
- **D**isability
- **E**xposure

The primary assessment is a *hands-on* evaluation. This contrasts with the general assessment, which is based only on what you see and hear in the first seconds that you encounter the child. In the primary assessment you assess the ABCDEs to categorize the type and severity of the child's clinical condition. Based on the category, you then decide the best action to take. This assessment includes evaluating vital signs and oxygen saturation by pulse oximetry. You will also perform a rapid test of blood glucose if needed.

> *Important:* During each step of the primary assessment, *watch for any life-threatening problem.* If one is present, call for help and start emergency support before you complete the rest of the assessment.

Once the primary assessment is completed and life-threatening problems are addressed, an advanced provider will usually perform the secondary and tertiary assessments.

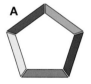

Airway

Airway Assessment

Assess the airway to decide if it is open and unobstructed (ie, patent):

- Look for movement of the chest or abdomen
- Listen for breath sounds and air movement
- Feel movement of air at the nose and mouth

Is the airway clear, maintainable, or not maintainable?

Status	Description
Clear	Airway is open and unobstructed for normal breathing
Maintainable	Airway can be maintained by *simple measures,* such as positioning or insertion of an oropharyngeal airway (OPA)
Not maintainable	Airway cannot be maintained without *advanced treatment*

Look for signs that suggest that the upper airway is obstructed:

- Increased inspiratory effort with chest retractions
- Abnormal inspiratory sounds (eg, snoring or high-pitched stridor)
- Decreased air movement despite increased respiratory effort

If the airway is obstructed, the next step is to decide if you can open and maintain the airway with *simple measures* or if you need to get help for *advanced treatment*.

Simple Measures

Simple measures to open and maintain upper airway patency may include one or more of the following:

Positioning	Allow the child to assume a position of comfort or position the child to open the airway. • If no injury is suspected, place the unresponsive child on her side. • Extend the child's neck and lift her chin. • If the older child is alert, allow him to sit up and lean forward in a "sniffing" position. • Elevate the head of the bed.
Head tilt–chin lift or jaw thrust	• Use a head tilt–chin lift to open the airway unless you suspect cervical spine injury. • If you suspect that a *cervical spine injury* is present, open the airway using a jaw thrust *without* head tilt. • If a jaw thrust does not open the airway, use a head tilt–chin lift or head tilt with a jaw thrust, because opening the airway is a priority. When giving CPR to a child with a possible cervical spine injury, manually stabilize the child's head and neck rather than using immobilization devices. (Note that the jaw thrust may be used in children without injury as well.)
Suctioning	Suction the nose and oropharynx.
FBAO relief techniques	Relieve foreign-body airway obstruction (FBAO) if the child is responsive: • If the child is <1 year of age: give back slaps and chest thrusts. • If the child is 1 year of age or older: give abdominal thrusts.
Airway adjuncts	Use airway adjuncts (eg, insert OPA)

Advanced Treatment

The child may need advanced treatment to maintain the airway. Advanced providers perform these interventions, which may include one or more of the following:

- Placing an advanced airway (eg, endotracheal tube)
- Removing a foreign body; this may require looking at the airway with a laryngoscope
- Applying continuous positive airway pressure (CPAP) or noninvasive positive-pressure breathing assistance
- Creating a surgical opening through the skin into the trachea

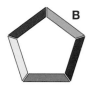

Breathing

Breathing Components

Assess breathing by evaluating

- respiratory rate
- respiratory effort
- air movement
- airway and breath sounds
- pulse oximetry

Respiratory Rate (Normal)

Normal breathing takes little work: breathing is quiet, with easy inspiration and passive expiration. The child will look comfortable. The normal respiratory rate is typically faster in infants and younger children and slower in older children (Table 1).

Table 1. Normal Respiratory Rates by Age[3]

Age	Breaths per Minute
Infant (<1 year)	30 to 60
Toddler (1 to 3 years)	24 to 40
Preschooler (4 to 5 years)	22 to 34
School age (6 to 12 years)	18 to 30
Adolescent (13 to 18 years)	12 to 16

 A respiratory rate that is consistently >60 breaths per minute in a child of any age is abnormal. This rate is a warning sign.

Try to evaluate the child's respiratory rate before you touch him. If the child becomes anxious or upset, his respiratory rate will often change. The respiratory rate may also be higher than normal if the child is ill or injured. Several conditions cause increased heart rate, including fever, excitement, anxiety exercise, or pain.

To determine the respiratory rate per minute, double the number of chest rises counted in 30 seconds. Be aware that normal sleeping infants may start and stop breathing in intervals of up to 10 to 15 seconds. If you count chest rises for less than 30 seconds, you may not estimate the rate accurately. Count the respiratory rate several times as you assess and reassess the child to detect changes. Alternatively you can continuously monitor the respiratory rate by using a cardiorespiratory monitor.

Be careful to consider the child's clinical condition when you evaluate the respiratory rate.

- A decrease in respiratory rate from fast to a more "normal" rate may indicate overall improvement. The child who is improving will have a better level of consciousness. She will also have reduced signs of air hunger and work of breathing.

- A decreasing or irregular respiratory rate may also indicate that the child's clinical condition is worsening. The child's general appearance or signs of circulation will often change as the child gets worse. Skin color may become pale, mottled, or cyanotic. The child's level of consciousness may decrease.

Respiratory Rate (Abnormal)

Abnormal respiratory rates are classified as

- fast
- slow
- apnea

Fast Respiratory Rate

A fast respiratory rate is a breathing rate that is faster than normal for age. This is often the first sign of respiratory distress in infants. It can also occur with stress.

A fast respiratory rate may be seen with signs of increased work of breathing. A fast respiratory rate, however, may also be seen *without* signs of increased work of breathing. This may result from

- conditions that do not involve the respiratory system, such as high fever, pain, and sepsis
- dehydration

Slow Respiratory Rate

A slower-than-normal respiratory rate may be caused by

- fatigue
- a central nervous system injury that affects the respiratory control center
- very low blood oxygen concentration (ie, low oxygen saturation by pulse oximetry)
- infection (usually serious)
- hypothermia
- drugs that depress the respiratory drive

 A slow respiratory rate or an irregular respiratory rate in a severely ill or injured infant or child is a serious sign. It often signals that the child may soon develop respiratory arrest.

Apnea

Apnea is a pause in breathing. The term *apnea* is used if there is no inspiratory airflow for at least 20 seconds. *Apnea* may also be used to describe a pause in inspiratory airflow of <20 seconds if other signs of inadequate breathing are present. Other signs of inadequate breathing can include slow heart rate, cyanosis, or pallor.

Respiratory Effort

Evaluate respiratory effort to assess the severity of the child's condition and the need for urgent action. The following are signs of increased respiratory effort:

- Nasal flaring
- Chest retractions
- Head bobbing or seesaw respirations

Other signs of increased respiratory effort are prolonged inspiratory or expiratory times, open mouth breathing, gasping, and use of accessory muscles. Grunting is a serious sign. Grunting may indicate severe respiratory distress or respiratory failure. See "Grunting" later in this section.

The child who has increased respiratory effort is trying to improve the level of oxygen in the body (oxygenation), to eliminate carbon dioxide (ventilation), or both. Increased respiratory effort can result from the following:

Causes	Clinical Conditions
Conditions that increase resistance to airflow	Asthma, bronchiolitis
Conditions that cause the lungs to be stiffer and difficult to inflate	Pneumonia, accumulation of fluid in the lungs or pleural space
Conditions that do not involve the respiratory system	Diabetic ketoacidosis (DKA), aspirin poisoning or other poisonings, other metabolic diseases

Nasal Flaring

Nasal flaring is enlargement of the nostrils with each inspiratory breath. The nostrils enlarge to maximize airflow during breathing. Nasal flaring is most commonly seen in infants and younger children. It is usually a sign of respiratory distress.

Chest Retractions

Chest retractions are an inward movement of the sternum or the soft tissues of the chest during inspiration. The retractions may be seen between the ribs, above or below the sternum. In more severe cases retractions may involve the entire chest wall. Chest retractions are a sign of increased respiratory effort. The child is using chest muscles to try to move air into the lungs. Air movement, however, is impaired by narrowing of the airways or by stiff lungs. Retractions may occur in several areas of the chest. The severity of the retractions generally corresponds with the severity of respiratory distress.

The table below describes the location of retractions commonly seen with each level of breathing difficulty:

Breathing Difficulty	Location of Retraction	Description
Mild ↓ Severe	Subcostal	Retraction of the abdomen, just below the rib cage
	Substernal	Retraction of the abdomen, at the bottom of the breastbone
	Intercostal	Retraction between the ribs
	Supraclavicular	Retraction in the neck, just above the collarbone
	Suprasternal	Retraction in the chest, just above the breastbone
	Sternal	Retraction of the sternum toward the anterior spine

Signs that accompany retractions are often clues to the cause of the child's condition:

- Retractions with stridor or an inspiratory snoring sound suggest upper airway obstruction.*
- Retractions with forced exhalation and expiratory wheezing suggest marked lower airway obstruction* (asthma or bronchiolitis) causing obstruction during both inspiration and expiration.
- Retractions with grunting or labored breaths suggest lung tissue disease.*

*Note: See Part 3: "Recognition of Respiratory Distress and Failure" for more information about these conditions.

Severe chest retractions may also be accompanied by head bobbing or seesaw respirations.

Head Bobbing or Seesaw Respirations

Be alert for other signs of increased respiratory effort. Two signs are head bobbing and seesaw respirations. These signs often mean that the child has severe respiratory distress and may get worse. If you see these signs, you should get help.

- Head bobbing is the use of the neck muscles to help the breathing effort. When the child breathes in, he lifts his chin and extends his neck. When he breathes out, his chin falls forward. Head bobbing is most frequently seen in infants. It can be a sign of respiratory failure.
- Seesaw respirations are a distinct form of "abdominal breathing." When the child breathes in, the chest retracts and the abdomen expands. When the child breathes out, the movement reverses: the chest expands and the abdomen moves inward. Note that normal infants can demonstrate "abdominal breathing," with the abdomen rising during inspiration. With normal breathing, however, the infant has no signs of increased respiratory effort.

Air Movement	To assess air movement, you should

- look for chest wall movement
- listen to breath sounds with a stethoscope (auscultate) for air movement

Chest Wall Movement

Chest expansion (chest rise) during inspiration should be equal (symmetrical) on both sides of the chest. Expansion may be subtle during spontaneous quiet breathing when the chest is covered by clothing. But chest expansion should be easy to see when the chest is uncovered. In normal infants the abdomen may move more than the chest during inspiration. Some causes of decreased or unequal chest expansion are

- inadequate effort
- airway obstruction
- aspiration of a foreign body
- collapse of all or part of the lungs
- thick secretions that block the airways
- collection of air, blood, or other fluid in the space surrounding the lungs

Breath Sounds

It is important to try to listen to breath sounds from the lower airways. Listen to the following areas:

Area	Location
Anterior	Mid chest (just to the left and right of the sternum)
Lateral	Under the armpits (the best location for evaluating air movement into the lower airways)
Posterior	Both sides of the back

Compare breath sounds in one area with sounds heard over other areas. You may hear normal breath sounds over some parts of the chest and abnormal sounds over others.

Listen to the loudness of breath sounds:

- Inspiratory sounds should be soft and quiet. Watch the movement of the child's chest as he tries to breathe in. These sounds should occur at the same time as the movement.
- Expiratory breath sounds are often short and even quieter. You may not even hear normal expiration sounds.

Note the quality of air movement. Because the child's chest wall is thin, it is easy to hear lung sounds from one part of the chest when your stethoscope is over another part of the chest. You may also hear breath sounds from the upper airway when you listen all over the chest. This is because sound is easily transmitted through the chest from the upper airway.

Sometimes the child's work of breathing and coughing suggests lower airway obstruction, but you don't hear wheezes. This may mean that the child is not breathing enough air to create wheezing and needs help.

You may have difficulty hearing breath sounds at all in a child who is obese. In this case it will be especially difficult to identify abnormalities. Assess the child's respiratory effort to look for signs of distress.

Abnormal Airway and Breath Sounds

During the primary assessment you should evaluate the child for abnormal airway and breath sounds. Abnormal sounds include stridor, grunting, gurgling, wheezing, and crackles.

Stridor

Stridor is a coarse, higher-pitched sound. It is typically heard during inspiration. Sometimes stridor may be heard on both inspiration and expiration. Stridor is a sign of upper airway obstruction (ie, located outside the chest). It may indicate critical airway obstruction requiring immediate action.

There are many causes of stridor:

Causes	Clinical Conditions
Infection	Croup
Congenital airway abnormalities	Laryngomalacia (collapse of the larynx)
Acquired airway abnormalities	Tumor, cyst, or weakness in one or both vocal cords
Upper airway edema	Allergic reaction or swelling after a medical procedure
Aspiration of foreign-body	Foreign-body airway obstruction

Grunting

Grunting is typically a short, low-pitched sound heard during expiration. Sometimes it may sound like a small cry, but it is present with almost every expiration. Grunting may accompany the child's response to pain or fever. Grunting is typically a sign of severe respiratory distress or failure from lung tissue disease. If grunting is present, get help.

Grunting can result from the following causes[4]:

Causes	Clinical Conditions
Pulmonary conditions	Pneumonia, acute respiratory distress syndrome, bleeding into the lungs
Cardiac conditions causing accumulation of fluid in the lungs	Inflammation of heart muscle, congestive heart failure
Abdominal conditions causing pain and abdominal splinting	Bowel obstruction, perforated bowel, appendicitis, inflammation of abdominal cavity

 Grunting occurs as the child exhales against partially closed vocal cords. Infants and children often grunt to open the small airways and air sacs in the lungs. This is an effort to improve oxygenation and ventilation.

Gurgling

Gurgling is a bubbling sound heard during inspiration or expiration. It occurs when the upper airway is obstructed by airway secretions, vomit, or blood.

Prolonged Expiration

Prolonged expiration is an increase in the time it takes the child to exhale. It is usually a sign of lower airway obstruction.

Wheezing

Wheezing is a high-pitched or low-pitched whistling or sighing sound heard most often during expiration. It occurs less frequently during inspiration. This sound indicates lower airway obstruction (ie, located inside the chest), especially of the smaller airways. Bronchiolitis and asthma are common causes of wheezing. Inspiratory wheezing suggests a foreign body or other cause of obstruction in the trachea or upper airway.

Crackles

Crackles are also known as rales. These are sharp, crackling sounds heard on inspiration. Crackles may be described as moist or dry:

- Moist crackles indicate accumulation of fluid in the air sacs. Moist crackles can be a sign of pneumonia or accumulation of fluid in the lungs.

- Dry crackles are heard more often with small airway collapse and diseases of the lung tissue surrounding the air sacs. The sound of dry crackles can be described as the sound made when you rub your hair together close to your ear.

Pulse Oximetry

Pulse oximetry is a tool used to monitor the percentage of the child's hemoglobin that is saturated with oxygen. This noninvasive method can detect low oxygen saturation in a child before it causes cyanosis or bradycardia.

The pulse oximeter consists of a probe attached to the child's finger, toe, or ear lobe. The probe is linked to a unit that displays the percent of hemoglobin that is saturated with oxygen. Many units also show the heart rate and beep with each pulse beat. Some models display the quality of the pulse signal as a waveform.

Monitor oxygen saturation readings to decide the best action:

Oxygen Saturation Readings	Action
Equal to or greater than 94% when breathing room air	Usually indicates adequate oxygenation; validate by clinical assessment
Less than 94% (hypoxemia) when breathing room air	Consider giving oxygen
Less than 90% in a child receiving 100% oxygen by a nonrebreathing mask (severe hypoxemia)	Call for help; additional actions are usually required

Interpreting Pulse Oximetry Readings

It is important to recognize that pulse oximetry indicates only the oxygen saturation of hemoglobin. It does not evaluate

- oxygen content of the blood (ie, how much oxygen is carried by the blood)
- oxygen delivery to the tissues

For example, if a child is profoundly anemic, oxygen saturation may be 100%, but oxygen delivery may be low.

> *If the heart rate on the pulse oximeter is not the same as the heart rate on the ECG monitor, the oxygen saturation reading is not reliable. Evaluate the child's circulation immediately. Also look at signs such as respiratory rate, respiratory effort, and level of consciousness.*

Unreliable Readings in Carbon Monoxide Poisoning

In a child with carbon monoxide poisoning, the pulse oximeter cannot tell the difference between

- hemoglobin saturated with carbon monoxide
- hemoglobin saturated with oxygen

This may result in a *falsely* high or normal oxygen saturation reading.

See Respiratory Resources on the student CD for a complete discussion of pulse oximetry.

Circulation

Circulation Assessment

To assess circulation, you will need to evaluate circulatory function by evaluating

- heart rate
- pulses (both peripheral and central)
- capillary refill time
- skin color and temperature
- blood pressure

The child's level of consciousness will help you evaluate blood flow to the brain. Urine output can also help you evaluate blood flow to the kidneys.

Circulatory Function

Heart Rate: Normal

Heart rate should be appropriate for the child's age, level of activity, and clinical condition (Table 2). Note the wide range for normal heart rate. Heart rate may also vary in a sleeping child or a child who is athletic. A child with a fever, especially a high fever, should have a faster heart rate.

> Get help if a child's heart rate is outside the normal range.

Table 2. Normal Heart Rates (per Minute) by Age

Age	Awake Rate	Average	Sleeping Rate
Newborn to 3 months	85 to 205	140	80 to 160
3 months to 2 years	100 to 190	130	75 to 160
2 years to 10 years	60 to 140	80	60 to 90
>10 years	60 to 100	75	50 to 90

Modified from Hazinski[3] and Gillette.[5]

To determine heart rate, check the pulse rate, listen to the chest, or view a monitor (ECG monitor or pulse oximeter). Attach a 3-lead ECG monitoring system when practical.

Abnormal Heart Rate

An abnormal heart rate is defined as either too fast (tachycardia) or too slow (bradycardia). Assess heart rate when the child is at rest.

Tachycardia

Tachycardia is a heart rate that is faster than the normal range for a child's age. A heart rate that is >200/min in infants or >180/min in children may be a sign of a life-threatening condition.

When the heart beats too fast, it has to work hard and may not fill completely with blood. This may result in inadequate blood flow. Tachycardia is a common, nonspecific sign of distress. It can develop in response to many problems. Tachycardia is often appropriate when the child is seriously ill or injured. However, tachycardia may indicate a rhythm problem.

Providers need information from the child's history, physical examination, and ECG analysis to determine the type of tachycardia. Sinus tachycardia and tachycardia from an abnormal rhythm are 2 types of tachycardia seen in children.

Sinus tachycardia is a rapid heart rate that originates in the natural pacemaker of the heart. It occurs in response to many problems. These problems include anxiety, exertion, fear, exercise, pain, and fever. Other problems are low oxygen delivery (eg, anemia), respiratory distress or failure, and dehydration. Sinus tachycardia may be a sign of heart disease or other serious illness. If a child has sinus tachycardia, quickly assess for shock and respiratory distress or failure.

Tachycardia from an abnormal rhythm may cause shock, heart failure, or even cardiac arrest.

Bradycardia

Bradycardia is a heart rate that is slower than normal for a child's age. When the heart beats too slowly, the heart may not pump enough blood flow to the major organs. Bradycardia may be normal in athletic children, but it can be a worrisome sign. Bradycardia with low blood pressure or poor circulation is never normal. Bradycardia may indicate that the child may soon be in cardiac arrest.

The most common causes of bradycardia in a child are respiratory distress and inadequate oxygen in the blood.

If the child with bradycardia ...	then ...
has decreased responsiveness or other signs of poor circulation	immediately support ventilation and provide oxygen. Be prepared to start chest compressions if needed.
is alert and responsive	consider other causes of slow heart rate, such as heart block or drug overdose. Note that a slow heart rate may be normal in athletic children.

Pulses

Evaluation of pulses is an important part of the assessment of circulation. Feel both the central and peripheral pulses.

In healthy infants and children (unless the child is obese or in a cold environment), you should be able to palpate the following pulses easily:

Central Pulses	Peripheral Pulses
Femoral	Brachial
Carotid (in older children)	Radial
Axillary	Dorsalis pedis
	Posterior tibial

Central pulses will be stronger than peripheral pulses. This is because these blood vessels are larger and closer to the heart. The difference in quality between central and peripheral pulses is exaggerated with the constriction of blood vessels seen in shock.

In shock, blood flow (ie, circulation) often decreases. The decrease in circulation starts in the arms and legs with loss of peripheral pulses. It then extends toward the trunk with eventual weakening of central pulses. A cold environment can constrict the blood vessels. This constriction can cause a difference in volume between peripheral and central pulses. Central pulses, however, should remain strong.

> *Weakening of central pulses is a worrisome sign that requires very rapid action to prevent cardiac arrest. Call for help and support airway, oxygenation, and breathing. Be prepared to give a fluid bolus or other support of the circulation.*

Capillary Refill Time

Capillary refill time is the time it takes for blood to return to tissue after you blanch it with pressure. Normal capillary refill time is 2 seconds or less. Capillary refill reflects circulation to the skin. Abnormalities in capillary refill may indicate problems with cardiac output.

To evaluate capillary refill, lift the arm or leg slightly above the level of the heart. It is best to evaluate capillary refill in an environment that is neither hot nor cold.

Frequent causes of delayed or prolonged capillary refill (a refill time >2 seconds) include

- dehydration
- shock
- hypothermia

Children with normal capillary refill time may still have shock. For example, children with "warm" septic shock may have a rapid (ie, <1 second) capillary refill time.

Skin Color and Temperature

Monitor changes in skin color and temperature (as well as capillary refill time) over time to assess a child's response to therapy. Skin color should be consistent over the trunk, arms, and legs. The mucous membranes, nail beds, palms of the hands, and soles of the feet should be pink. Skin temperature should be warm.

When blood flow decreases, the hands and feet are typically affected first. They may become cool, pale, dusky, or mottled. If the condition worsens, the skin over the trunk, arms, and legs will also become cool with poor color.

 Consider the temperature of the child's environment when assessing skin color and temperature. If the environment is cool, the child may have cool skin with poor color even though circulation is good. Mottling or pallor with cool skin may be present. Capillary refill may be delayed, particularly in the fingers, legs, and toes.[6]

To assess skin temperature, use the back of your hand, which is more sensitive to temperature changes than the palm, which has thicker skin. Slide the back of your hand up the arm or leg to see if there is a point where the skin temperature changes from cool to warm. Monitor this area between the warm and cool skin over time. Changes will give information about the child's response to therapy. The point should move down the limb as the child's condition improves.

Carefully evaluate *pallor, mottling,* and *cyanosis,* which may indicate inadequate oxygen delivery to the tissues.

Pallor

Pallor, or paleness, is a lack of normal color in the skin or mucous membranes. Causes of pallor include

- decreased blood flow to the skin (can be caused by cold, stress, hypovolemic shock)
- decreased number of red blood cells (anemia)
- decreased skin pigmentation

Pallor does not necessarily indicate disease; it can result from lack of sunlight or inherited paleness.

> *Look at the mucous membranes: lips, lining of the mouth, tongue, lining of the eyes. If the child has pale mucous membranes or pale palms and soles, look for other signs of shock.*

Pallor is often difficult to detect in a child with dark or thick skin. Family members often can tell you if a child's color is abnormal. Pallor of the lips and mucous membranes strongly suggests anemia or very poor circulation (shock).

Mottling

Mottling, or mottled skin, is an irregular or patchy discoloration of the skin. When mottling is present, some irregular skin areas are pink while others may appear pale or cyanotic. Mottling may occur as a result of

- variations in skin coloring
- shock
- decreased oxygen saturation in the blood

Shock and a decrease in oxygen saturation in the blood results in an irregular supply of oxygenated blood to the skin. It can even produce cyanosis in some areas. Some conditions that can cause this are low blood levels of oxygen (caused by a respiratory problem), low blood volume, or shock.

Cyanosis

Cyanosis is a bluish discoloration of the skin and mucous membranes. Blood saturated with oxygen is bright red, but blood that does not carry as much oxygen is dark bluish-red. Cyanosis may be easier to see in the mucous membranes and nail beds, particularly in children with darker skin. It can also appear on the feet, nose, and ears. Cyanosis may be caused by low blood flow (shock, a circulatory problem) or low levels of oxygen in the blood (a respiratory problem).

Note if the cyanosis is

- peripheral cyanosis—seen over hands and feet
- central cyanosis—seen in mucous membranes (eg, inside the mouth)

If you see cyanosis, you need to get help.

> *A child who develops central cyanosis typically needs emergency actions, such as oxygen and support of ventilation.*

Blood Pressure

To measure blood pressure accurately, you must use a properly sized cuff. The cuff bladder should cover about 40% of the circumference of the mid-upper arm.[7] The blood pressure cuff should extend at least 50% to 75% of the length of the upper arm.

Normal Blood Pressures

Table 3 lists normal blood pressure values by age and gender. Like heart rate, there is a wide range of values within the normal range.

Table 3. Normal Blood Pressures in Children by Age

Age	Systolic Blood Pressure (mm Hg)		Diastolic Blood Pressure (mm Hg)	
	Female	**Male**	**Female**	**Male**
Neonate (1st day)	60 to 76	60 to 74	31 to 45	30 to 44
Neonate (4th day)	67 to 83	68 to 84	37 to 53	35 to 53
Infant (1 mo)	73 to 91	74 to 94	36 to 56	37 to 55
Infant (3 mo)	78 to 100	81 to 103	44 to 64	45 to 65
Infant (6 mo)	82 to 102	87 to 105	46 to 66	48 to 68
Infant (1 y)	68 to 104	67 to 103	22 to 60	20 to 58
Child (2 y)	71 to 105	70 to 106	27 to 65	25 to 63
Child (7 y)	79 to 113	79 to 115	39 to 77	38 to 78
Adolescent (15 y)	93 to 127	95 to 131	47 to 85	45 to 85

This table summarizes the range from the 33rd to 67th percentile in the first year of life and from the 5th to 95th percentile for systolic and diastolic blood pressure according to age and gender and assuming the 50th percentile for height for children 1 year of age and older. Blood pressure ranges taken from the following sources: Neonate, Infant (1 to 6 mo)[8]; Infant (1 y), Child, Adolescent.[9]

Hypotension

Hypotension is defined by the following thresholds of systolic blood pressure (Table 4).

Table 4. Definition of Severe Hypotension by Systolic Blood Pressure and Age

Age	Systolic Blood Pressure (mm Hg)
Term neonates (0 to 28 days)	<60
Infants (1 to 12 months)	<70
Children 1 to 10 years 5th blood pressure percentile	<70 + (age in years × 2)
Children >10 years	<90

Note that these blood pressure values will overlap with normal blood pressure values for about 5% of healthy children.

If a child's systolic blood pressure falls 10 mm Hg from baseline, immediately evaluate the child for additional signs of shock. In addition, remember that these threshold values are based on studies of normal, resting children. Children with injury and stress will typically have high blood pressure. Blood pressure in the low-normal range may indicate a problem in a seriously ill or injured child.

 Hypotension in the child represents severe shock when the child can no longer maintain normal blood pressure. (Tachycardia and constriction of the blood vessels are some mechanisms that the body uses to maintain normal blood pressure.)

Hypotension may be a sign of septic shock. In this condition the main problem is excessive dilation (relaxation and enlargement) of the blood vessels.

A child with a fast heart rate and low blood pressure may develop a *slow* heart rate when his condition worsens. This is a sign of a life-threatening problem. You should call for help. Support airway, breathing, and oxygenation. The child will need urgent support of the circulation, such as administration of a fluid bolus.

Circulation to the Brain and Kidneys

Brain

Clinical signs of brain function are important signs of overall blood flow and oxygen delivery in the ill or injured child. These signs include level of consciousness, muscle tone, and pupillary responses to light.

Low oxygen delivery in the brain that is severe or occurs suddenly may produce the following neurologic signs:

- Decrease in muscle tone
- Seizures
- Pupil dilation
- Loss of consciousness

You may observe other signs when oxygen delivery to the brain declines gradually. These signs can be subtle and are best detected with repeated measurements over time:

- Change in level of consciousness with confusion
- Irritability
- Lethargy
- Agitation alternating with lethargy

 Changes in neurologic signs may be caused by conditions other than low levels of oxygen delivery to the brain. Some drugs and metabolic conditions (eg, high ammonia levels) or increased intracranial pressure (ICP) may produce neurologic signs and symptoms. Thus, you should not assume that altered brain function is just due to low oxygen delivery to the brain. Instead, look for other signs of low blood flow (shock) as the cause of the signs you observed.

The child's neurologic condition may be characterized using the Alert–Voice–Painful–Unresponsive (AVPU) scale and a description of pupil responses. The AVPU Pediatric Response Scale and pupil responses are reviewed in the section on disability assessment.

Kidneys

Adequate urine output usually indicates adequate blood flow to the kidneys. Normal urine output varies with age.

Normal urine output in well-hydrated infants, young children, older children, and adolescents is as follows:

Age	Normal Urine Output
Infants and young children	1.5 to 2 mL/kg per hour
Older children and adolescents	1 mL/kg per hour

Initial urine output that drains immediately after a catheter is inserted represents the amount of urine currently held in the bladder. After that initial volume, the amount of urine collected over time reflects ongoing urine production. If the child has no known kidney disease and suddenly has a decrease in urine output, you should suspect that the child has low blood volume or other causes of shock. If urine output is low because of hypovolemic shock, it should improve if you administer adequate fluid.

 High amounts of glucose in the blood spill into the urine carrying water with it. This results in increased urine output and high amounts of glucose in the urine. Blood glucose concentration is easy to detect using a bedside glucose test. Glucose in the urine is easy to detect using a test strip.

#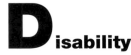

Disability Assessment

The disability assessment is a quick evaluation of 2 main components of the central nervous system: the cerebral cortex and the brainstem. As you perform the general and primary assessments, you should note the child's response and activity.

> *As a child's level of consciousness decreases, the child will progress from irritability to agitation to anxiety to decreased responsiveness. These are important clues to the child's clinical condition.*

Formal disability evaluation is often completed at the end of the primary assessment. Repeat it to monitor for changes in the child's neurologic status. Standard evaluations include

- AVPU Pediatric Response Scale
- response of pupils to light
- blood glucose test

AVPU

To rapidly evaluate cerebral cortex function, use the AVPU Pediatric Response Scale.[10] This scale is a system for rating a child's level of consciousness. The level of consciousness is an indicator of cerebral cortex function. The scale consists of 4 ratings:

A	Alert	The child is awake, active, and responds appropriately to parents and external stimuli. "Appropriate response" is assessed based on the child's age and the setting or situation.
V	Voice	The child responds only when you or the parents call the child's name or speak loudly.
P	Painful	The child responds only to a painful stimulus, such as rubbing the breastbone with your knuckles.
U	Unresponsive	The child does not respond to any stimulus.

Causes of a decreased level of consciousness in children include

- decreased blood flow to the brain, such as from increased ICP or severe shock
- brain injury
- infection in the brain (eg, encephalitis or meningitis)
- hypoglycemia (low blood sugar)
- drug overdose
- low blood levels of oxygen

> *If the child demonstrates a change in level of consciousness or if she suddenly does not respond to stimulation, call for help. Immediately support airway, breathing, and circulation as needed.*

Response of Pupils to Light

Response of pupils to light is a useful indicator of brainstem function. *If pupil response is abnormal, the child needs advanced life support.*

Normally pupils constrict in response to light and dilate in a dark environment. Be sure to use a bright light. If the pupils do not constrict in response to direct light stimulus (eg, flashlight directed at the eyes), a brainstem injury may be present. The pupils are generally equal in size, but slight variations are normal. Irregularities in pupil size or response to light may occur as a result of eye injury or other conditions.

During the disability assessment, record the following for each eye:

- Size of pupils (diameter in millimeters)
- Equality of pupils (right = left; right greater than left; left greater than right)
- Constriction of pupils to light (ie, the speed of the pupil response to light and the size when constricted)

The acronym PERRL (**P**upils **E**qual **R**ound **R**eactive to **L**ight) describes the normal responses of pupils.

Blood Glucose Test

You should monitor the blood glucose level of any seriously ill infant or child. Low blood glucose level may cause altered level of consciousness and other signs. It can cause brain injury if it is not quickly recognized and adequately treated. Measure blood glucose level with a rapid bedside glucose test.

For more information about the recognition and treatment of hypoglycemia, see Part 6: "Management of Shock."

E

Exposure

Introduction

Exposure is the final component of the primary assessment. When the child is seriously ill or injured, you should measure the child's core temperature. In addition, you should undress the child as appropriate to permit a focused physical examination. Remove clothing as necessary one area at a time. If you suspect the child has a spine injury, use your hands to stabilize the child's head and neck when you turn the child.

Carefully assess the child's face, trunk (front and back), arms, and legs. If you detect significant hypothermia, begin warming measures.

During this part of the exam, look for evidence of injury or trauma. Examples are bleeding, burns, or unusual marks that might be caused by abuse. Feel the arms and legs. Note the child's response. If there is obvious tenderness to touch, that area may be injured. You may need to immobilize the arm or leg.

You may see petechiae and purpura, which are purple discolorations in the skin that do not blanch with pressure. They are caused by bleeding from capillaries and small vessels and often represent a serious or life-threatening problem, such as infection.

Type of Purple Skin Discoloration	Appearance	Suggests
Petechiae	Tiny dots	Low platelet count
Purpura	Larger spots	Septic shock

Secondary Assessment

Brief Summary

The secondary assessment consists of a focused medical history using the SAMPLE mnemonic and a thorough physical examination. SAMPLE stands for

- **S**igns and Symptoms
- **A**llergies
- **M**edications
- **P**ast medical history
- **L**ast meal
- **E**vents leading to presentation

See the *PALS Provider Manual* for a detailed discussion of the secondary assessment.

Tertiary Assessment

Brief Summary

The tertiary assessment includes laboratory, radiographic, and other tests to help find the cause or severity of the child's problem. The term *tertiary* means that these tests are a third way to assess the child. It does not mean that these tests are third in order of performance. The tests are performed based on the child's condition. See the *PALS Provider Manual* for a detailed discussion of the tertiary assessment.

Life-Threatening Conditions

Signs of a Life-Threatening Condition

If you detect a life-threatening problem at any time during your assessment, get help. You should also support the child's airway, breathing, and circulation. Signs of a life-threatening condition may include the following:

Airway	Complete or severe airway obstruction
Breathing	Apnea, slow respiratory rate, very fast respiratory rate, significant work of breathing
Circulation	Tachycardia, bradycardia, absence of detectable pulses, poor blood flow, hypotension
Disability	Decreased response or abnormal motor response (posturing) to pain, unresponsiveness
Exposure	Significant hypothermia, petechiae/purpura consistent with septic shock, significant bleeding, abdominal distention consistent with an acute abdomen

Actions

Start lifesaving actions immediately and get help if

- the patient has a life-threatening condition
- you are uncertain or "something feels wrong"

If the child does not have a life-threatening condition, advanced providers can start secondary and tertiary assessments. These assessments are summarized in the *PALS Provider Manual*.

Part ③

Recognition of Respiratory Distress and Failure

Overview

Introduction

It is easy to see if a child is breathing or not breathing. It is more difficult to decide if a child

- is working hard to breathe and is in respiratory distress
- is getting worse and is in respiratory failure

When you categorize the type and severity of the child's respiratory problem, you will be able to decide the best actions to take.

Some respiratory problems will improve with simple measures, such as giving oxygen. Other conditions require immediate action using more advanced airway treatments, such as insertion of an advanced airway.

The goal is to stop the progression from respiratory distress so that the child does not develop respiratory failure, respiratory arrest, and then cardiac arrest. This can happen quickly in infants and children. The survival rate after respiratory arrest is higher than the survival rate after cardiac arrest. Once the child is in cardiac arrest, outcome is generally poor.

> *The earlier you detect respiratory distress or respiratory failure and start appropriate therapy, the better chance the child has for a good outcome.*

Learning Objectives

After completing this part you should be able to

- define respiratory distress and respiratory failure
- recognize the signs of respiratory distress and respiratory failure
- recognize the signs of inadequate oxygenation and inadequate ventilation
- recall the 4 types of respiratory problems and recognize the signs and symptoms of each

Factors Associated With Respiratory Problems

In order to recognize respiratory distress or failure, you need to understand a few basic factors associated with respiratory problems. This section discusses decreased oxygenation and ventilation in respiratory problems.

Decreased Oxygenation and Ventilation in Respiratory Problems

Function of the Respiratory System

The main function of the respiratory system is to exchange gases. Oxygen is taken into the lungs during inspiration. It moves from the lung air sacs (alveoli) into the blood and attaches to hemoglobin. Carbon dioxide moves from the blood into the air sacs. Carbon dioxide leaves the body during expiration. Acute respiratory problems can result from any airway, lung tissue, or neuromuscular disease. These problems can cause low oxygen saturation, high levels of carbon dioxide (poor ventilation), or both.

Infants and children have high metabolic rates. This means that they need a high amount of oxygen for their body weight.

Respiratory problems may result in the following conditions:

Condition	Term
Low oxygen saturation of the arterial blood	Hypoxemia
Inadequate ventilation leading to increased carbon dioxide levels in the blood	Hypercarbia
Both low oxygen saturation and high carbon dioxide concentration	Both hypoxemia and hypercarbia

Low Oxygen Saturation (Hypoxemia)

Low oxygen saturation is called *hypoxemia*. When hypoxemia is present, the hemoglobin saturation with oxygen (often called the oxygen saturation) is low. Normally hemoglobin in the arteries is fully saturated (100% saturated) with oxygen. You can detect low oxygen saturation by using pulse oximetry.

An oxygen saturation of <94% in a normal child breathing room air indicates hypoxemia.

In many children a low oxygen saturation in the blood will cause a low tissue level of oxygen (hypoxia). This can cause the child's condition to quickly worsen. Hypoxemia is only one cause of tissue hypoxia.

 Some children with low oxygen saturation (eg, children with cyanotic heart disease) may be able to deliver enough oxygen to the tissues even though they are hypoxemic.

Signs of Low Oxygen Saturation (Hypoxemia)

Signs of hypoxemia are

- fast respiratory rate
- slow respiratory rate, apnea (late)
- signs of increased respiratory effort: nasal flaring, chest retractions, head bobbing, seesaw respirations
- tachycardia (early)
- bradycardia (late)
- pallor
- mottling
- cyanosis (late)
- agitation, anxiety (early)
- decreased level of consciousness (late)

Inadequate Ventilation (Hypercarbia)	If the child's ventilation is inadequate the child will develop high levels of carbon dioxide in the blood. This condition is called *hypercarbia*. Causes of hypercarbia are

- decreased respiratory effort
- airway obstruction (upper or lower)
- lung tissue disease

> *Hypoxemia is easy to detect using pulse oximetry. Hypercarbia, however, is more difficult to detect. This is because many of the clinical signs of hypercarbia are the same as the signs of hypoxemia. To confirm that the child has high carbon dioxide levels in the blood, the advanced provider may obtain a blood sample for blood gas analysis.*

Monitoring for Inadequate Ventilation and Hypercarbia	It is very important to watch for signs of inadequate ventilation. The clinical signs of inadequate ventilation and hypoxemia may be identical. When a child presents with hypoxemia, give oxygen. If oxygen saturation increases but signs of increased respiratory effort or decreased level of consciousness are present, the child may be developing hypercarbia. You should get help.

Decreased level of consciousness is an important clue that the child's ventilation may not be adequate. If hypoxemia is corrected when you give oxygen but the child's level of consciousness worsens, the child's carbon dioxide level is probably increased. With worsening hypercarbia, the child's level of consciousness often deteriorates from agitation and anxiety to decreased responsiveness.

Categorize Respiratory Problems by Severity

Respiratory Distress

Definition	Respiratory distress is a clinical state of

- increased respiratory rate
- increased respiratory effort (work of breathing)

A child in respiratory distress may also have changes in air movement, airway and breath sounds, oxygen saturation, skin color, and level of consciousness.

Clinical Characteristics of Respiratory Distress

Respiratory distress ranges from mild to severe.

A child with ...	has ...
a normal level of consciousness *and* • good air movement *and* • mild increase in respiratory rate *or* • mild increase in respiratory effort *or* • changes in airway and breath sounds	mild respiratory distress

A child with ...	has ...
a decreased level of consciousness *or* • marked increase in respiratory rate *or* • significant increase in respiratory effort *or* • decreased air movement *or* • poor skin color	severe respiratory distress*

*Severe respiratory distress may indicate respiratory failure.

Respiratory distress is apparent when a child tries to maintain adequate gas exchange despite respiratory problems. As the child tires or as respiratory function or effort decreases, signs of respiratory failure develop.

Clinical Signs of Respiratory Distress

Clinical signs of respiratory distress may vary in severity. Typical signs of respiratory distress include some or all of the following:

- Increased respiratory rate
- Increased respiratory effort
- Abnormal airway and breath sounds (eg, stridor, wheezing, grunting)
- Tachycardia
- Pale, cool skin
- Changes in level of consciousness

Respiratory Failure

Definition

Respiratory failure is defined as inadequate oxygenation, ventilation, or both. If respiratory failure is present, you must act to prevent respiratory arrest and ultimately cardiac arrest.

Clinical Characteristics of Respiratory Failure

If the child with respiratory distress does not improve or worsens, respiratory failure is probably present. It may be caused by upper or lower airway obstruction, lung tissue disease, or disordered control of breathing. Examples of disordered control of breathing are periods of apnea or shallow, slow respirations.

Some children with respiratory failure may not have signs of increased respiratory effort. This happens in cases of disordered control of breathing. *When respiratory effort is inadequate, respiratory failure may occur without typical signs of respiratory distress.*

A child's condition may be categorized as probable respiratory failure based on clinical findings. Laboratory tests may be required to confirm respiratory failure.

Clinical Signs of Respiratory Failure

Some signs of probable respiratory failure are

- very fast respiratory rate—early
- slow respiratory rate, irregular breathing rate or apnea—late
- increased, decreased, or no respiratory effort
- decreased air movement
- tachycardia—early
- bradycardia—late
- cyanosis
- altered level of consciousness

Categorize Respiratory Problems by Type

Introduction

There are 4 types of respiratory problems:

- Upper airway obstruction
- Lower airway obstruction
- Lung tissue disease
- Disordered control of breathing

Respiratory problems do not always occur one at a time. A child may have more than 1 type of respiratory problem. For example, a child may have disordered control of breathing due to a head injury. She may then develop pneumonia (lung tissue disease).

Upper Airway Obstruction

Obstruction of the upper airways (ie, the airways outside the chest) may occur in the nose, pharynx, or larynx. Obstructions can range from mild to severe. Common causes of upper airway obstruction are the following:

Upper Airway Obstruction	Common Causes
Tongue blocking the airway	Reduced level of consciousness
Foreign-body aspiration	Aspiration of food or a small object
Swelling of the tissues lining the upper airway	Allergic reaction, tonsil enlargement, croup, or epiglottitis
Mass narrowing the airway lumen	Abscess or tumor
Thick secretions obstructing the nasal passages	Infection
Congenital airway abnormality narrowing the airway	Complete tracheal rings

Upper airway obstruction also may be caused by a medical treatment or procedure. For example, narrowing of the airway below the vocal cords may develop as a result of injury to the tissues during endotracheal intubation.

Clinical Signs of Upper Airway Obstruction

Clinical signs of upper airway obstruction include general signs of increased respiratory rate and effort. Signs are seen most often during *inspiration*. The following are common signs:

Common Signs of Upper Airway Obstruction
Increased respiratory rate
Increased respiratory effort: inspiratory chest retractions, nasal flaring
Decreased air movement: poor chest rise, poor air entry when you listen with a stethoscope
Stridor: typically inspiratory
Seal-like cough
Snoring or gurgling during inspiration
Change in voice: hoarseness

Note if respiratory effort, air movement, or airway and breath sounds change over time. Sometimes an infant or child can begin with partial airway obstruction and develop complete airway obstruction. When the obstruction is complete, chest retractions and effort increase, and inspiratory sounds disappear. You will hear little or no air movement with a stethoscope.

The child may have other signs, such as drooling, seesaw breathing, or cyanosis. With upper airway obstruction, the respiratory rate is often only mildly elevated. This is because a rapid respiratory rate increases the work of breathing.

Lower Airway Obstruction

Obstruction of the lower airways (ie, the airways within the chest) may occur in the lower trachea, the bronchi, or the bronchioles. Asthma and bronchiolitis are common causes of lower airway obstruction.

Clinical Signs of Lower Airway Obstruction

Clinical signs of lower airway obstruction include general signs of increased rate and effort. These signs are seen most often during *expiration*. Common signs of lower airway obstruction are as follows:

Common Signs of Lower Airway Obstruction
Increased respiratory rate
Increased respiratory effort: chest retractions, nasal flaring
Decreased air movement
Prolonged expiratory phase: expiration is an active rather than a passive process
Wheezing: heard most commonly on expiration; may also occur on both inspiration and expiration. Inspiratory wheezes alone are uncommon.

Lung Tissue Disease

Lung tissue disease is a term given to a group of problems that affect lung function. With lung tissue disease, the air sacs and small airways of the lungs are collapsed or filled with fluid. They no longer contain an air-oxygen mixture. Because oxygen isn't moving from the air sacs into the blood, children with lung tissue disease have reduced oxygen saturation in the blood. With severe lung tissue disease, ventilation is also reduced. This causes the level of carbon dioxide in the blood to rise. The lungs are often heavy and may become stiff, so the child's work of breathing increases.

Lung tissue disease has many causes. They are

- pneumonia from any cause: bacterial, viral, fungal, chemical
- accumulation of fluid in the lungs associated with congestive heart failure or leaking of fluids into the tissues (eg, sepsis, acute respiratory distress syndrome)
- trauma (eg, lung bruise)
- allergic reaction
- toxins

Clinical Signs of Lung Tissue Disease

The following are clinical signs of lung tissue disease:

Clinical Signs of Lung Tissue Disease
Increased respiratory rate (often marked)
Increased respiratory effort, especially during inspiration
Decreased air movement
Grunting
Crackles (rales)
Decreased breath sounds or change in pitch of breath sounds

Low oxygen saturation is usually present in lung tissue disease and may not respond to oxygen administration alone. Often other advanced support is needed.

Disordered Control of Breathing

Disordered control of breathing is an abnormal, usually slow breathing pattern. Symptoms of inadequate respiratory rate, effort, or both are present. Often the parent will say the child is "breathing funny." This condition is often caused by a neurologic disorder. Some neurologic disorders that may affect breathing control are

- seizures
- central nervous system infection
- head injury
- brain tumor
- increased ICP
- hydrocephalus (increased accumulation of fluid surrounding the brain)
- neuromuscular disease

Clinical Signs of Disordered Control of Breathing

The following are clinical signs of disordered control of breathing:

Clinical Signs of Disordered Control of Breathing	
Sign	**Characteristic**
Variable respiratory rate	Fast or normal rate alternating with slow rate, periods of apnea
Variable respiratory effort	Increased work of breathing alternating with decreased work of breathing, periods of absent respiratory effort
Air movement	Normal or decreased
Normal breath sounds or snoring sounds	Produced by the tongue falling back into the airway, causing upper airway obstruction

Shallow breathing often causes inadequate oxygenation and ventilation. Disordered control of breathing is usually caused by a condition that impairs brain function. For this reason children with disordered control of breathing often have a decreased level of consciousness.

Management of Respiratory Distress and Failure

Overview

Introduction

Respiratory problems are a major cause of cardiac arrest in children. It may be very hard to decide if a child is in respiratory distress or respiratory failure based on clinical signs. In children respiratory problems can rapidly get worse. Thus, there is little time to waste when deciding what actions to take.

> If respiratory problems are treated promptly, the child has a better chance of survival. If a child in respiratory arrest progresses to cardiac arrest, the outcome is generally poor. For the best outcome, you must act quickly to restore respiratory function.

This part discusses actions to take for children in respiratory distress and failure.

Learning Objectives

After completing this part you should be able to

- describe actions to stabilize the child with respiratory distress and respiratory failure
- discuss specific actions for management of upper airway obstruction, lower airway obstruction, lung tissue disease, and disordered control of breathing
- explain the use of pulse oximetry and describe its limitations

Initial Management of Respiratory Distress and Failure

Introduction

The primary goal for initial management of a child in respiratory distress or failure is to support or restore adequate oxygenation and ventilation. You build on your *assessment* of airway and breathing to *categorize* the type and severity of the respiratory problem. Based on this categorization, you *decide* what to do. First, *act* to support oxygenation and ventilation. Then repeat the "assess-categorize-decide-act" approach to decide the next best actions to take.

Initial Management of Respiratory Distress and Failure

For a child in respiratory distress or failure, initial management may include the actions listed in Table 5. Of course, the actions that you take will be based on your scope of practice and local protocols.

> You should get help or seek expert consultation when caring for an infant or child with moderate or severe respiratory problems.

Table 1. Initial Management of Respiratory Distress or Failure

Assess	Action (as indicated)
Airway	• Support the airway (allow the child to assume a position of comfort) or position the child to open the airway (perform manual airway maneuvers). – If you suspect that the child may have a cervical spine injury, open the airway using a jaw thrust without head extension. If this maneuver does not work, use a head tilt with either chin lift or jaw thrust. Remember that opening the airway is a priority if airway obstruction is present. • Clear the airway (suction nose and mouth as indicated; remove a foreign body if you see it). • Insert an OPA as indicated.
Breathing	• Assess oxygenation and ventilation. • Assist ventilation (eg, bag-mask ventilation) if needed. • Give oxygen. Provide humidified oxygen if available. Use a high-flow/high-concentration oxygen delivery system for severe respiratory distress or respiratory failure if available. • Monitor oxygen saturation by pulse oximetry. • Monitor respiratory rate and effort. • Give medication as needed (eg, albuterol, nebulized epinephrine).
Circulation	• Monitor heart rate (note that the pulse oximeter will provide a continuous display). • Monitor level of consciousness. • Ensure vascular access as needed (for fluid therapy and medications). • If the child has poor circulation, consider giving 20 mL/kg intravenous (IV) isotonic crystalloid (normal saline [NS] or lactated Ringer's [LR]).

> *Remember the ACDA approach: perform frequent reassessment.*

Actions Based on the Cause of the Problem

Decide what actions to take for a child in respiratory distress or failure based on the cause (category) of the problem.

This part discusses specific actions to take for the following 4 types of respiratory problems:

- Upper airway obstruction
- Lower airway obstruction
- Lung tissue disease
- Disordered control of breathing

Management of Upper Airway Obstruction

Introduction

Upper airway obstruction is a block in the large airways outside the chest. It may range from mild to severe. Common causes are

- an aspirated foreign body
- tissue swelling (above, at, or below the vocal cords)
- decreased level of consciousness resulting in the tongue obstructing the airway

Several factors can contribute to airway compromise in infants and children:

- A child's tongue is large in proportion to his mouth and throat. It is a common cause of upper airway obstruction.
- An infant's head is large in proportion to his body. If an infant lies face up on his back, his neck is more likely to flex. This causes his neck to tilt forward and adds to the obstruction caused by the tongue.
- The upper airway is smaller in infants and young children. It is more easily obstructed. Infection, inflammation, or injury can cause secretions or blood in the airways, nose, pharynx, and larynx. Airway obstruction can result.

General Management of Upper Airway Obstruction

General management of upper airway obstruction includes the initial actions listed in Table 5. Additional measures focus on relieving the obstruction. These measures may include opening the airway by

- removing any object that you see obstructing the airway
- suctioning the nose, mouth, or both
- reducing airway swelling using drugs, such as nebulized epinephrine
- allowing the child to assume a position of comfort
- avoiding unnecessary agitation, which often worsens upper airway obstruction
- deciding if an airway adjunct or advanced airway is needed
- deciding early if a surgical airway is needed

Suction the airway if blood or secretions are present. *Use caution, however, if the cause of upper airway swelling is an infection (eg, croup). In many of these patients, blind suctioning is relatively contraindicated. Suctioning produces increased agitation. This increases respiratory distress.* Instead allow the infant or child to assume a position of comfort. Give nebulized epinephrine if there is swelling of the airway below the tongue.

If you recognize severe upper airway obstruction, *call for advanced help.* The provider with the greatest skills and experience in airway management is most likely to successfully establish an airway. Failure to aggressively treat an acute upper airway obstruction may lead to complete airway obstruction and ultimately cardiac arrest.

In less severe cases of upper airway obstruction, infants and children may benefit from specific airway adjuncts. An OPA should be inserted in only an unconscious patient. In the conscious child an OPA stimulates gagging and may cause vomiting.

Specific Actions Based on the Cause of the Upper Airway Obstruction

Some causes of upper airway obstruction may require specific actions. This section gives actions to take for upper airway obstruction due to the following common causes:

- Croup
- Anaphylaxis
- Other obstructions (eg, foreign-body airway obstruction, abscess)

Actions to Take for Croup

Decide which actions to take for croup based on your assessment of severity.[11] General actions for upper airway obstruction include the initial actions described in Table 5. *Specific actions for croup* may include the actions described below.[11-17]

Severity	Signs	Actions
Mild croup	• Occasional barking cough • Limited to no stridor at rest • Few to no chest retractions	May give cool mist
Moderate croup	• Frequent barking cough • Audible stridor • Retractions at rest • Little to no agitation • Good distal air entry on auscultation • Decreased oxygen saturation	• Get help • Administer humidified oxygen • Keep NPO • Administer nebulized epinephrine • Observe for at least 2 hours after giving epinephrine for "rebound" (recurrence of stridor)
Severe croup	• Frequent barking cough • Prominent inspiratory stridor • Occasional expiratory stridor • Marked chest retractions • Decreased air entry on auscultation • Significant agitation • Decreased oxygen saturation	
Impending respiratory failure	• Weak cough • Audible stridor at rest (can be difficult to hear with failing respiratory effort) • Chest retractions (may not be marked with failing respiratory effort) • Decreased air movement on auscultation • Lethargy or decreased level of consciousness • Cyanosis unless oxygen is administered	• Get help • Assist ventilation (ie, bag-mask ventilation) • Administer a high flow/high concentration of oxygen; use a nonrebreathing mask if assisted ventilation is unnecessary • Administer nebulized epinephrine

Actions to Take for Anaphylaxis

Decide what actions to take for anaphylaxis based on your assessment of the severity of the allergic reaction.

Mild allergic reaction

Signs of a mild allergic reaction are

- stuffy nose, sneezing, and itching around the eyes
- itching of the skin
- raised, red rash on the skin (hives)

Actions for Mild Allergic Reaction
Get help.
Look for medical alert identification on the child.

Severe allergic reaction

The signs of a severe allergic reaction are

- trouble breathing
- swelling of the tongue and face
- fainting

In addition to the general actions described in Table 5, *specific actions for a severe allergic reaction* may include the actions described below.[18-20]

Action
The first and most important action in the child with moderate to severe airway obstruction due to anaphylaxis is to give epinephrine. • Give IM epinephrine by autoinjector. (Give a pediatric dose if the child's weight is 10 to 30 kg. Give an adult dose if weight is 30 kg or greater.)
• Get help.
• If wheezing is present, give albuterol by metered-dose inhaler (MDI) or nebulizer solution.
• Give continuous nebulization if indicated (e, severe wheezing).
If hypotension is present: • Administer isotonic crystalloid (eg, NS or LR) 20 mL/kg IV bolus.

Actions to Take for Other Obstructions

In addition to the general actions described in Table 5, *specific actions for other obstructions* (eg, foreign-body airway obstruction, abscess) may include the actions described below.

Action
Get help. Provide initial support. In cases of *mild to moderate upper airway obstruction* where the child is still breathing effectively: • Allow the child to assume a position of comfort (mild to moderate upper airway obstruction, responsive child) • Administer oxygen in high flow/high concentration as tolerated; use a nonrebreathing mask if available *If the child has more severe symptoms:* • Perform a jaw thrust or head tilt–chin lift (severe or complete upper airway obstruction, poorly responsive or unresponsive child) • Get help immediately from an appropriately skilled provider (eg, anesthesiologist or otolaryngologist)

(Continued)

Action

If the child is unable to breathe adequately and you suspect a foreign body (complete or severe upper airway obstruction), try to remove the foreign body as follows:
 	
• For a conscious infant or child, use manual techniques appropriate for the child's age:
  – <1 year: back slaps and chest thrusts
  – 1 year or older: abdominal thrusts
 	
• If the child becomes unconscious, look in the mouth and remove any visible object. Open the airway and try to provide bag-mask ventilation. If you cannot give effective ventilation despite several attempts, start cycles of compressions and attempted ventilation (even if a palpable pulse is present) until advanced life support providers are available. Before you give breaths after a cycle of chest compressions, look in the child's mouth and remove any visible object. Chest compressions may help move the object so it no longer obstructs the airway.
 	
Note: Do not perform a *blind finger sweep* to relieve a foreign-body airway obstruction. This technique may push the foreign body further into the airway. It could also cause injury and bleeding.

Attempt ventilation (ie, bag-mask ventilation) as indicated; may require high inflating pressures—if so, disable the pop-off valve if present; consider using the 2-person bag-mask ventilation technique.
Administer nebulized racemic epinephrine or L-epinephrine as indicated (eg, stridor).

Management of Lower Airway Obstruction

Introduction

Lower airway obstruction involves mild or severe block of the airways inside the chest, such as the bronchi and bronchioles. Common causes are bronchiolitis and asthma.

General Management of Lower Airway Obstruction

General management of lower airway obstruction includes the initial actions described in Table 5.

In infants or children with respiratory failure or severe respiratory distress, the priority is restoring adequate oxygenation. Correction of inadequate ventilation (hypercarbia) is not as important. Children typically tolerate inadequate ventilation without adverse effects as long as tissue oxygen delivery is adequate. Thus, you will focus on supporting adequate oxygen saturation.

If assisted ventilation is required for lower airway obstruction, perform *bag-mask ventilation at a relatively slow respiratory rate.*

Providing ventilation at a slow rate allows more time for expiration. This reduces the risk that air will remain inside the chest at the end of expiration. If you give too many breaths or breaths that are too large, you will prevent the heart from refilling with blood. This can decrease blood flow. If you use a slow respiratory rate, you can lengthen the inspiratory time to prevent high airway pressure.

High airway pressure can result in the following complications:

Complication	Result
Air enters the stomach (gastric distention)	• Increased risk of vomiting and aspiration • Can prevent normal movement of the diaphragm, limiting effective ventilation
Risk of air leak into space surrounding the lungs	• Decreased blood flow • Risk of lung collapsing from air leaking into the pleural space (pneumothorax)
Severe air trapping	• Severe decrease in oxygenation • Decreased blood flow

Specific Actions Based on Cause of Lower Airway Obstruction

Some causes of lower airway obstruction require specific actions. This section gives actions to take for lower airway obstruction due to the following common causes:

- Bronchiolitis
- Acute asthma

Note: It may be difficult to decide if a wheezing infant has bronchiolitis or asthma. A history of previous wheezing episodes suggests that the infant has asthma. Consider giving bronchodilators if the diagnosis is unclear.

Actions to Take for Bronchiolitis

In addition to the general actions described in Table 5, *specific actions for bronchiolitis* may include the following:

Action
Perform oral or nasal suctioning as needed.
Assist ventilation with bag-mask as indicated.

The results from clinical trials are mixed regarding the use of bronchodilators for bronchiolitis.[21-23] The following are findings:

- Some infants respond to nebulized epinephrine or albuterol.
- In a few studies nebulized epinephrine has been shown to improve symptoms better than albuterol.[24-26]
- Some infants get worse after nebulizer therapy.

You may give nebulized epinephrine or albuterol based on local protocol or as directed by an advanced provider. Discontinue treatment if there is no benefit or if the child gets worse.

Actions to Take for Acute Asthma

In addition to the general actions described in Table 5, *specific actions for acute asthma* may include the actions described below.[27-32]

Decide what actions to take for asthma based on your assessment of the clinical severity. Severity of asthma is classified as mild, moderate, or severe (Table 6). Also watch for signs that a child with asthma is getting worse:

- Decreased wheezing with continued increased effort
- Decreased oxygen saturation
- Decreased level of consciousness

Table 2. PEARS Modified Asthma Severity Score: Classification of Mild, Moderate, and Severe Asthma*

Parameter[†]	Mild Asthma	Moderate Asthma	Severe Asthma	Respiratory Arrest Imminent
Alertness	May be agitated	Usually agitated	Usually agitated	Drowsy or confused
Positioning	Can lie down	Prefers sitting	Hunched forward	
Breathless	Walking	Talking (infant will have softer, shorter cry; difficulty feeding)	At rest (infant will stop feeding)	
Talks in	Sentences	Phrases	Words	
Respiratory rate	Increased	Increased	Increased	
Respiratory effort	Usually not increased	Usually increased	Usually increased	Seesaw respirations
Wheezing	Moderate (often only end-expiration)	Loud	Usually loud	Absent
Pulse oximetry (SpO$_2$ room air)	>95%	91% to 95%	<90%	
Heart rate	Normal to increased	Increased	Increased	Decreased

*Modified from National Heart, Lung, and Blood Institute and World Health Organization: Global Strategy for Asthma Management and Prevention NHLBI/WHO Workshop Report, US Department of Health and Human Services, Revised September 1997. Publication no. 97-4051.

[†]The presence of several parameters, but not necessarily all, indicates the general classification of the attack.

Severity of Asthma	Action
Mild to moderate	• Get help. • Give oxygen by nasal cannula or blow-by oxygen; if needed, give high-flow/high-concentration humidified oxygen; adjust based on child's oxygen saturation. • Give albuterol by MDI or nebulizer solution.
Moderate to severe	• Get help. • Give high-flow/high-concentration humidified oxygen to keep oxygen saturation >90%; use a nonrebreathing mask if needed. • Give albuterol by MDI or nebulizer solution. • May give other drugs such as nebulized ipratropium bromide and corticosteroids as directed by an advanced provider. • Consider establishing vascular access for administration of fluids or medications.
Impending respiratory failure	• Get help. • Administer high-flow/high-concentration oxygen; use a nonrebreathing mask if available. • Assist ventilation (ie, bag-mask ventilation) as indicated. • Give albuterol by MDI or nebulizer solution. • May give other drugs such as nebulized ipratropium bromide and corticosteroids as directed by an advanced provider. • Establish vascular access for administration of fluids and medications.

Management of Lung Tissue Disease

Introduction

Lung tissue disease is a category of respiratory problems that affect lung function. Lung tissue disease has many causes. One is infectious pneumonia. This condition results from inflammation at the level of the air sacs. The inflammation can be caused by bacteria, viruses, or fungi.[33] Other causes include fluid in the lungs, trauma, allergic reaction, and toxins.

Management of Lung Tissue Disease

General management of lung tissue disease includes the initial actions described in Table 5. If the child is wheezing or if there is evidence of airway obstruction, actions may include giving a bronchodilator. Monitor clinical signs of circulation. Support as necessary.

If the child has lung tissue disease due to infectious pneumonia, consider the following actions:

Action
Get help.
Begin antibiotic therapy quickly after drawing blood cultures.
Administer albuterol by MDI or nebulizer solution if wheezing is present.
If the child has fever, take measures to reduce the temperature.

Management of Disordered Control of Breathing

Introduction	Disordered control of breathing is an abnormal breathing pattern. This pattern is a *variable* one: the child will have a normal or fast respiratory rate alternating with a slow rate or periods of apnea.
Treatment of Disordered Control of Breathing	General management of disordered control of breathing includes the initial actions described in Table 5. Priorities are opening the airway, suctioning secretions if present, and supporting ventilation.

Often the child with disordered breathing will require an advanced airway. Immediately call for help when you recognize this condition. Give bag-mask ventilation to stabilize the child until advanced providers arrive. Further therapy depends on the underlying cause.

Common causes of disordered control of breathing are

- increased ICP
- poisoning or drug overdose
- neuromuscular disease |
| **Increased ICP** | Increased ICP can complicate a variety of conditions involving the brain. These conditions include inflammation, infection, bleeding, trauma, tumor, and accumulation of fluid surrounding the brain.

An irregular respiratory pattern can be a sign of increased ICP. The combination of irregular breathing or apnea, a rise in blood pressure, and bradycardia suggests a marked increase in ICP. Children with increased ICP, however, often have tachycardia rather than bradycardia, with irregular breathing and increased blood pressure. |
| **Poisoning or Drug Overdose** | One of the most common causes of respiratory failure following a poisoning or drug overdose is depression of control of breathing. A less common cause is weakness or paralysis of respiratory muscles.

Frequent complications of disordered breathing in this setting are

- upper airway obstruction
- poor respiratory rate and effort
- low oxygen saturation
- aspiration of stomach contents or oral secretions into the lungs
- respiratory failure

Complications from a depressed level of consciousness include pneumonia due to aspiration or accumulation of fluid in the lungs because of lung injury. These complications may result in respiratory failure. |
| **Neuromuscular Disease** | Chronic neuromuscular disease affects the muscles of respiration. Children with these diseases commonly take very shallow breaths and do not have a strong cough. As a result they may develop complications. Examples are collapse of the small airways and airway sacs (lung tissue), stiff lungs, and pneumonia. Chronic respiratory distress and respiratory failure are other complications. |

Additional Actions to Take Based on Cause

Actions to take for these specific causes of disordered control of breathing include those in Table 5. Other actions you should take in addition to those in Table 5 are as follows:

Cause	Action
Increased ICP	• Get help. • Elevate the child's head; keep in midline. • Treat fever. • Assist ventilation to provide hyperventilation. (*Note:* Avoid hyperventilation in most circumstances. If you suspect that the child has a critical increase in ICP, however, use hyperventilation to help stabilize the child until advanced providers take over the care of the child.)
Poisoning or drug overdose	• Get help. • If you suspect poisoning, contact your local poison control center. (In the United States call 1-800-222-1222.) For more information on toxicology, see Part 10.2 of the *2005 AHA Guidelines for CPR and ECC*. • Be prepared to suction the airway if vomiting occurs.
Neuromuscular disease	• Get help. • Suctioning the mouth is often helpful; the child with neuromuscular weakness often has a weak cough and can't keep the upper airway clear.

Part 5

Recognition of Shock

Overview

Introduction

Early recognition and treatment of shock is a key to improving outcome in critically ill or injured children. If left untreated, shock can quickly progress to cardiopulmonary failure and then to cardiac arrest. Once the child is in cardiac arrest, outcome is poor.

This part discusses the following topics:

- The effect of severity of shock on blood pressure (compensated versus hypotensive shock)
- Causes and signs of the 4 types of shock

Once you *categorize* the child's shock based on type and severity, then you *decide* which lifesaving actions to provide. These *actions* are discussed in Part 6: Management of Shock.

> *If you recognize shock quickly and start therapy, you increase the child's chance for a good outcome.*

Learning Objectives

After completing this part you should be able to

- define shock
- describe how to evaluate signs of circulation
- recall the types of shock (hypovolemic, distributive, cardiogenic, and obstructive)
- differentiate between compensated shock and hypotensive shock
- recognize clinical signs and symptoms of shock

Definition of Shock

Introduction

Shock is a critical condition that results when the tissues do not get as much oxygen as they need. Children in shock often, but not always, have inadequate blood flow.

The definition of shock does not depend on blood pressure. Shock may occur with

- normal blood pressure
- increased blood pressure
- decreased blood pressure

For most children in shock, the amount of blood (blood flow) pumped by the heart is low. Some children in shock, however, have a higher-than-normal blood flow. High blood flow is often seen in sepsis or in the child with severe anemia. All forms of shock can result in impaired function of vital organs, such as

- the brain: decreased level of consciousness
- the kidneys: low urine output, decreased kidney function

Causes of Shock

Shock can result from the following causes:

Causes of Shock	Types of Shock
Inadequate blood volume	Hypovolemic shock, including hemorrhage
Inappropriate distribution of blood flow	Distributive/septic shock
Impaired pumping of the heart	Cardiogenic shock
Obstructed blood flow	Obstructive shock

Any problems that cause the tissues to need more oxygen can make shock worse. Some of these conditions are fever, infection, injury, respiratory distress, and pain.

The important point to remember is that in shock *tissues are not getting as much oxygen as they need to function,* whether it is because of

- not enough oxygen delivery to the tissues
- increased demand of the tissues for oxygen

When the tissues are starved for oxygen, cell and organ damage can occur. This damage may not be reversible. Death may rapidly result from shock or later from organ failure.

> *The treatment goal for shock is to restore blood flow to the tissues. This prevents organ injury. It may also halt the progression to cardiopulmonary failure and cardiac arrest.*

Categorize Shock by Severity (Effect on Blood Pressure)

Introduction

The severity of shock can be categorized by its effect on systolic blood pressure.

Compensated shock	The child's systolic blood pressure is normal.
Hypotensive* shock	The child's systolic blood pressure is lower than normal (hypotension).

*Hypotensive shock was previously referred to as "decompensated" shock.

Categorizing the severity of shock as compensated or hypotensive does not capture the variations of severity. It does, however, provide a simple way to recognize when very rapid actions are needed.

Recognizing the Severity of Shock

The severity of shock may range from mild to moderate to severe. Hypotensive shock is easy to recognize when you measure blood pressure. Compensated shock may be more difficult to recognize. The signs and symptoms of shock are affected by the

- type of shock
- cause of shock

Remember, severe shock may occur with normal or low blood pressure. In some cases children with low systolic blood pressure will still maintain adequate blood flow to meet tissue demand. On the other hand, some children with normal blood pressure may have severe shock. These children will have other symptoms such as absent pulses and decreased level of consciousness.

You should *not* rely on a blood pressure reading alone to categorize severity of shock. Make decisions based on the entire assessment. Keep these important points in mind:

- Automated blood pressure devices are accurate only when the child has adequate circulation to the arms and legs. If you cannot palpate peripheral pulses and the arms and legs are cool with delayed capillary refill, an automated blood pressure reading may not be reliable.

- If blood pressure measurement is not available, evaluate other signs of circulation. Assess heart rate, peripheral and central pulses, capillary refill time, and skin color and temperature.

- Infants and children with compensated shock may be critically ill with severe shock despite a "normal" systolic blood pressure.

Note that in compensated shock, the *systolic* pressure is normal, but the *diastolic* pressure may be abnormal (ie, low or high).

Compensated Shock

If the child has normal systolic blood pressure but has signs of poor circulation, the child is in compensated shock. In this stage of shock the body is still able to maintain adequate blood pressure and blood flow to the brain and the heart. The body reduces blood flow to organs like the skin and kidneys and redirects it to the brain and heart. These changes in blood flow produce some of the signs of shock. The signs vary according to the type and severity of shock.

During your assessment of a seriously ill or injured child, look for signs of shock (Table 7).

Table 1. Common Signs of Shock

Area	Sign
Heart	Tachycardia
Skin	Cold, pale, mottled (in septic shock may be bright red) Delayed capillary refill Sweating
Pulses	Weak peripheral pulses
Kidney	Decreased urine output
Brain	Agitation, anxiety

Signs specific to the cause of shock are discussed later in this part.

Hypotensive Shock

The child has hypotensive shock if the following are present:

- Systolic hypotension
- Signs of poor circulation

Hypotension develops when attempts to maintain systolic blood pressure and blood flow are no longer effective. One key clinical sign that a child's condition is getting worse is a change in level of consciousness. This occurs when there is not enough blood flow to the brain. Hypotension is a late finding in most types of shock. Unless rapidly corrected, it may be a sign that shock cannot be reversed or that cardiac arrest may occur soon.

Hypotension Formula

In children 1 to 10 years of age, hypotension is defined as a systolic blood pressure reading calculated as

$$<70 \text{ mm Hg} + [\text{child's age in years} \times 2] \text{ mm Hg}$$

See Table 4: Definition of Severe Hypotension by Systolic Blood Pressure and Age in Part 2.

Progression of Shock

You must be alert to signs that the child's condition is getting worse. If untreated, shock will progress from compensated shock to hypotensive shock and then to cardiac arrest. Warning signs include

- absence of peripheral pulses
- decrease in level of consciousness/responsiveness

Bradycardia and weak-to-absent central pulses usually mean that the child will soon be in cardiac arrest.

Accelerating Process

It may take hours for compensated shock to progress to hypotensive shock. It may take only minutes for hypotensive shock to progress to cardiopulmonary failure and cardiac arrest. The progression from compensated shock to hypotensive shock and then to cardiac arrest is typically an *accelerating process*.

Compensated Shock

Possibly hours

Hypotensive Shock

Potentially minutes

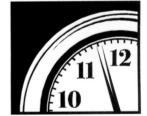

Cardiac Arrest

Act quickly to treat compensated shock. Your timely actions may prevent progression to hypotensive shock and cardiac arrest.

Categorize Shock by Type

Types of shock

Shock can be categorized into 4 basic types:

- Hypovolemic
- Distributive
- Cardiogenic
- Obstructive

Hypovolemic Shock

Hypovolemia is the most common cause of shock in children worldwide. Fluid loss due to diarrhea is the leading cause of hypovolemic shock. In fact, diarrhea and associated dehydration and electrolyte abnormalities are a major worldwide cause of infant death. Causes of hypovolemic shock include

- diarrhea
- hemorrhage (internal or external)
- vomiting
- inadequate fluid intake
- high urine output (eg, DKA)
- fluid leak into tissues as may occur with septic shock
- burns

The child with hypovolemic shock has decreased blood volume. You must quickly replace the fluid to stabilize the child in shock. To treat shock you often will have to give amounts of fluid by IV or IO infusion that are greater than the volume the child lost.

Signs of Hypovolemic Shock

Table 8 outlines typical signs of hypovolemic shock that you might see when evaluating the child during the general and primary assessments.

Table 2. Signs of Hypovolemic Shock

Primary Assessment	Sign
A	
B	• Increased respiratory rate • Normal or increased respiratory effort
C	• Tachycardia • Weak or absent peripheral pulses • Normal or weak central pulses • Delayed capillary refill • Cool to cold, pale, mottled, sweaty skin • Normal systolic blood pressure or hypotension • Decreased urine output
D	Changes in level of consciousness
E	

Distributive Shock

In distributive shock blood volume is not distributed appropriately. Some tissues receive too much blood flow, and other tissues do not receive enough blood flow.

The most common forms of distributive shock are

- septic shock
- anaphylactic shock
- neurogenic shock (eg, head injury, spinal injury)

Although septic, anaphylactic, neurogenic, and other types of distributive shock are not typically classified as hypovolemic shock, they all share a common characteristic. This characteristic is that blood is not distributed where it is needed. The child must receive IV fluids and cardiac drugs to support blood flow. The treatment goal is to increase blood flow to all tissues.

Another cause of the decrease in blood volume is fluid leaking from the blood vessels.

Signs of Distributive Shock

Table 9 outlines typical signs of distributive shock that you might see during the general and primary assessments of the child. The **boldface** text denotes type-specific signs that distinguish distributive shock from other forms of shock.

The high blood flow and widening of blood vessels often seen in distributive shock are the opposite of the low blood flow and narrowing of blood vessels seen in hypovolemic, cardiogenic, and obstructive shock.

In distributive shock diastolic blood pressure is typically lower than normal. Systolic blood pressure will also fall, especially if you don't give enough IV fluid therapy or you don't give it quickly.

Table 3. Signs of Distributive Shock

Primary Assessment	Finding
A	Usually patent unless level of consciousness is significantly impaired
B	• Fast respiratory rate • Normal respiratory effort or increased effort if the child has pneumonia, lung injury, or heart failure • Normal breath sounds or crackles
C	• Tachycardia • **Very strong peripheral pulses (bounding)** • **Warm flushed skin with brisk capillary refill (warm shock) or cool skin with delayed capillary refill (cold shock)** • Systolic and diastolic blood pressures may be normal, low, or high
D	• Changes in level of consciousness (agitation, confusion, or decreased responsiveness in late shock)
E	• Variable temperature (in sepsis may have low or increased temperature) • Petechial or purpuric rash (septic shock)

Septic Shock

Septic shock is the most common form of distributive shock. It is caused by the body's response to infectious organisms or their byproducts. These organisms stimulate the immune system and trigger the release of substances that cause inflammation.

In the early stages of sepsis there is an inflammatory response throughout the body. The illness progresses to septic shock in the late stages. The child's signs may evolve over days or take only hours. The clinical signs and progression vary widely. This continuum of events is called the septic cascade:

- The infectious organism or its byproducts activate inflammation.
- Inflammatory substances, known as cytokines, become active.
- Cytokines cause blood vessel walls to relax, which makes the blood vessels wider. Cytokines also cause fluids to leak into the tissue.
- Cytokines and other inflammatory products may also reduce the pumping function of the heart.

Widespread activation of inflammatory substances can lead to organ failure, particularly[34]

- decreased pumping function of the heart, widening of the blood vessels, and hypotension
- respiratory failure
- abnormal clot formation or bleeding
- decreased production of stress hormone

Causes	Effect
Decreased pumping function of the heart, wider blood vessels, and leaking of fluid into tissues	• Some tissues receive too much blood flow while other tissues receive too little • Skin may receive more blood flow than needed, causing the child to appear flushed (warm shock) • Hypotension
Inflammatory substances	• Decreased pumping function of the heart • Fever • Abnormal clot formation and/or bleeding
Decreased production of stress hormones	Decreased pumping function of the heart

Signs of Septic Shock

In the early stages, signs of septic shock may be difficult to detect. Circulation to the arms and legs may appear to be normal. Because septic shock is triggered by an infection or its byproducts, the child may also have

- fever or, less often, low temperature
- minor changes in level of consciousness (such as confusion)
- an elevated or decreased white blood cell count

In addition to the findings listed in Table 9, the child with septic shock may have petechiae or purpura.

Treatment Considerations

Because fluid is leaking into the tissues, you should anticipate that the child may develop fluid in the lungs when you give large amounts of IV fluid rapidly. Look for signs of respiratory distress. Recognize this potential complication, but do not let it prevent you from giving adequate fluid to restore blood flow.

Early recognition and treatment of septic shock are important to good outcome. You should identify signs of shock before hypotension develops. See "Management of Shock" for details on the treatment of septic shock.

Anaphylactic Shock

Anaphylactic shock results from a severe reaction to a drug, vaccine, food, toxin, plant, venom, or other antigen. This acute reaction often occurs seconds to minutes after exposure.

In anaphylactic shock the body releases substances that relax the blood vessels. This causes fluid to leak into the tissues. Bronchial tubes narrow, causing wheezing. Like septic shock, there is inappropriate distribution of blood volume.

The child needs support of the airway and breathing. In addition, you will need to give large amounts of IV fluid quickly. Death may occur rapidly after exposure, or the child may develop acute-phase signs that typically begin 5 to 10 minutes after exposure.

Signs and Symptoms

Signs and symptoms may include

- anxiety or agitation
- nausea and vomiting
- hives
- swelling of the face, lips, and tongue
- respiratory distress with stridor, wheezing, or both
- hypotension
- tachycardia

Hives are caused by histamine release. Swelling of the face, lips, and tongue may result in mild to severe upper airway obstruction. Wheezing is a sign of lower airway obstruction (bronchospasm). Hypotension is caused by hypovolemia due to widened blood vessels and fluid leaking into the tissues. Tachycardia is a sign that the body is trying to maintain blood flow to the tissues.

Neurogenic Shock

Neurogenic shock, including spinal shock, usually results from cervical spine (neck) injury. It may also be caused by a head injury or an injury to the spine above the level of the sixth thoracic (T6) vertebra. The injury disrupts the nerve supply to the blood vessels and the heart.

Physiology of Neurogenic Shock

The sudden loss of nervous system signals to smooth muscle in the vessel walls results in widening of the blood vessel walls.

Signs of Neurogenic Shock

Primary signs of neurogenic shock are

- hypotension with a low diastolic blood pressure
- normal heart rate or bradycardia

Unlike other forms of shock with low or normal blood pressure, *in neurogenic shock the heart rate is not fast.* This distinguishes neurogenic shock from the other forms of distributive shock.

Another sign is increased respiratory rate. During breathing the child may also use the muscles of the diaphragm instead of those in the chest wall.

The spine injury that causes spinal shock also injures the nerves to the skeletal muscles. You will see other signs of a high thoracic or cervical spine injury (eg, loss of movement or sensation).

It is important to understand the difference between hypovolemic shock and neurogenic shock.

Hypovolemic Shock	Neurogenic Shock
Hypotension	Hypotension
Tachycardia	Normal heart rate or bradycardia

Cardiogenic Shock

A child in cardiogenic shock has poor circulation resulting from decreased pumping function of the heart. This can be caused by pump failure (poor contractility), congenital heart disease, or rhythm abnormalities

Common causes of cardiogenic shock include

- congenital or genetic heart disease
- inflammation of the heart muscle
- abnormality of pumping function
- arrhythmias
- sepsis
- poisoning or drug toxicity
- injury to the heart (eg, trauma)

Signs of Cardiogenic Shock

Table 10 outlines typical signs of cardiogenic shock that you might see during the general and primary assessments of the child. The **boldface** text denotes type-specific signs that distinguish cardiogenic shock from other forms of shock.

Table 4. Findings Consistent With Cardiogenic Shock

Primary Assessment	Finding
A	
B	• Fast respiratory rate • Increased respiratory effort (chest retractions, nasal flaring) resulting from fluid in the lungs
C	• Tachycardia • Weak or absent peripheral pulses • Normal and then weak central pulses • Delayed capillary refill with cool arms and legs • Cold, pale, mottled, sweaty skin • **Cyanosis** • Normal or low blood pressure • Decreased urine output • **Signs of congestive heart failure (eg, fluid in the lungs, liver enlargement, distended neck veins)**
D	• Change in level of consciousness (agitation or anxiety early, reduced responsiveness later)
E	• Variable temperature

Reassessment of the Child in Cardiogenic Shock

For cardiogenic shock, oxygen saturation may be low if lung tissue disease is present.

> *A child with cardiogenic shock usually has a fast respiratory rate with increased respiratory effort. By comparison, a child in hypovolemic shock usually has a fast respiratory rate **without** increased respiratory effort.*

If a child has *cardiogenic* shock, you should not give large or rapid fluid boluses. The boluses can worsen fluid in the lungs. They may also worsen heart function. Remember the following:

- Give small isotonic fluid boluses (5 to 10 mL/kg).
- Give fluid boluses over longer periods of time (eg, 20 minutes instead of 5 to 10 minutes).
- Monitor the child closely during fluid infusion.

Infants and children with cardiogenic shock often require drug therapy to improve heart function and circulation. In addition, treatment includes methods to decrease oxygen needs. You should try to reduce the work of breathing and treat fever.

Obstructive Shock

Obstructive shock is a condition of low blood flow caused by a block in blood flow pathways. Types of obstructive shock include the following:

Cause	Type of Obstructive Shock
Accumulation of fluid in the sac around the heart	Cardiac tamponade
Accumulation of air outside the lungs in the chest cavity	Tension pneumothorax
Obstruction of normal blood flow from the heart as a result of congenital heart disease	Ductal-dependent lesions
Blood clot to the lungs	Pulmonary embolism

The obstruction to blood flow results in decreased blood flow to the tissues. As the condition progresses, increased respiratory effort, cyanosis, and signs of poor circulation become more apparent.

Treatment

The treatment of obstructive shock is cause-specific. Immediate recognition and correction of the underlying cause of the obstruction can be lifesaving.

> *If you think the child has obstructive shock, get help immediately. Without immediate treatment, children with obstructive shock often progress rapidly to cardiopulmonary failure and cardiac arrest.*

Obstructive shock is infrequent in children but may be seen in children with congenital heart disease or trauma. For more information see the *PALS Provider Manual*.

Part 6

Management of Shock

Overview

Introduction

Once you categorize shock in a seriously ill or injured child, immediate action can greatly improve outcome.

This part discusses goals of shock management and actions to take for a child in shock. It also includes information on fluid therapy and the importance of monitoring blood glucose.

Learning Objectives

After completing this part you should be able to

- describe the general goals of shock management
- summarize the initial priorities for stabilizing the child in shock
- describe effective principles of IV fluid therapy for shock
- explain how effective shock therapy depends on targeting the cause and degree of shock
- state the rate and volume of fluid administration for shock

Goals of Shock Management

Introduction

The goals in treatment of shock are to

- improve oxygen content in the blood
- improve blood flow to the tissues
- reduce tissue demand for oxygen
- support organ function
- prevent cardiac arrest

Immediate action for a child in shock may be lifesaving. The more time that passes between the event that caused the shock and the start of treatment, the worse the outcome. If the child with shock progresses to cardiac arrest, the outcome is generally poor.

Warning Signs

You must be alert to signs that the seriously ill or injured child is getting worse. Warning signs that the child is getting worse are

- marked tachycardia
- absent peripheral pulses
- weakening central pulses
- cold hands and feet with very prolonged capillary refill
- narrowing pulse pressure
- altered level of consciousness
- hypotension (late finding)

Once hypotension is present, organ damage may occur even if the child does not develop cardiac arrest.

> *Early recognition of compensated shock is critical to effective actions and good outcome.*

General Management of Shock

For a child in respiratory distress or failure, initial management may include the actions listed in Table 5. Of course, the actions that you take will be based on your scope of practice and local protocols.

Actions to Take for Shock

Deciding the best action to take and then acting quickly may be lifesaving for a child in shock.

> *You should get help or seek expert consultation when caring for an infant or child with shock.*

The following actions might be appropriate for a child in shock:

- Positioning
- Oxygen administration
- Support ventilation
- Vascular access
- IV fluid therapy
- Monitoring
- Frequent reassessment
- Get help

Note that 2 or more of these actions may be carried out at the same time.

Positioning

Positioning is important for a child in shock.

- Open and maintain the airway.
- Place a hypotensive child on her back. Raise her feet above the level of the heart. Make sure that breathing is not compromised.
- Allow a stable child to remain in her most comfortable position. For infants and young children, the best position might be in the arms of the parent or caregiver. This will help decrease anxiety and activity during the general and primary assessments.

Oxygen Administration

Be sure that the child has an open airway. Prepare to support the airway if necessary. Give humidified high-flow/high-concentration oxygen to all children in shock.

Support Ventilation	Assess respiratory rate and effort. Be prepared to support ventilation with bag mask as needed.

Vascular Access

Once you support airway and breathing, the next priority is to gain vascular access. Vascular access is needed for fluid therapy and drug administration. For children in compensated shock, peripheral venous access is preferred if it can be obtained rapidly. For children in hypotensive shock, immediate vascular access is critical. For these children, early IO access is encouraged. IO access should be used as soon as possible if needed in compensated or hypotensive shock.

For more information, see "Intraossecus Access" on the student CD.

IV Fluid Therapy

Once vascular access is established, give fluid boluses immediately.

> *Give isotonic crystalloid* in a 20 mL/kg bolus over 5 to 20 minutes to restore blood flow and blood pressure.*

Remember that if the pumping function of the heart is poor, you should give smaller fluid boluses (about 5 to 10 mL/kg) over the longer period of time (about 10 to 20 minutes).

As you give the fluid, monitor for

- development or worsening of fluid in the lungs
- increased respiratory effort
- decreased circulation

Be prepared to support oxygenation and ventilation if necessary.

*See "Isotonic Crystalloid Solutions" later in this part.

Monitoring

Assess the effectiveness of fluid resuscitation by frequent or continuous monitoring of

- oxygen saturation with pulse oximetry
- heart rate
- peripheral pulses
- capillary refill
- skin color and temperature
- blood pressure
- urine output
- level of consciousness
- blood glucose

Effective treatment will improve signs of circulation. The heart rate will decrease toward normal. Feel the quality of the peripheral pulses frequently. Monitor oxygen saturation and measure blood pressure as soon as practical. Insert a urinary catheter for accurate measurement of urine output. Assess level of consciousness and temperature.

Frequent Reassessment

Frequently reassess the child's breathing, circulation, and level of consciousness to

- evaluate trends in the child's condition
- determine response to therapy
- plan the next actions

At any point the child's condition could worsen and require lifesaving actions. Examples of lifesaving actions are opening the airway or providing assisted ventilation. Continue frequent reassessment until the child's condition is stable or the child is transferred to another level of care.

> *The condition of a child in shock is dynamic. Continuous monitoring and frequent reassessment are essential. This will help evaluate trends in the child's condition and determine response to therapy.*

Get Help

Remember that for specific categories of shock, lifesaving actions may be required that are beyond your scope of practice. Many of these actions are discussed in the *PALS Provider Manual*.

> *Sometimes the most important action that you can take for a child in shock is to get help. This includes calling a resuscitation code, activating the emergency response system, or alerting more advanced providers.*

Summary: General Management

Table 11 summarizes general management components discussed in this section.

> *Remember to get help or seek expert consultation when caring for an infant or child with shock.*

Table 11. Fundaments of Shock Management

Open and support the airway
Position the child • Stable: allow to remain with caregiver • Unstable: if hypotensive, place child on her back and raise the feet above the level of the heart unless breathing is compromised
Give a high flow/high concentration of oxygen
Support ventilation as needed
Ensure vascular (IV/IO) access • Consider IO access early (according to scope of practice)
Begin IV fluid therapy for shock • Give bolus (20 mL/kg) of isotonic crystalloid over 5 to 20 minutes. • Give a smaller volume (5 to 10 mL/kg) for bolus treatment and give over 10 to 20 minutes if poor heart function is present or suspected.
Start monitoring • Oxygen saturation by pulse oximetry • Heart rate by pulse oximetry and ECG monitor • Blood pressure • Urine output • Level of consciousness • Temperature
Perform frequent reassessment • Evaluate trends • Determine response to therapy
Get help

IV Fluid Therapy for Shock

Introduction

IV or IO fluid therapy is indicated for treatment of shock. The primary goal of fluid therapy is to restore blood flow to the tissues. The rate and volume of fluid therapy are affected by the cause of the condition. Rapid fluid therapy is used for hypovolemic and distributive shock. Other types of shock and conditions require adjustment of rate and volume.

Either isotonic crystalloid or colloid solutions may be used for fluid therapy. Blood and blood products generally are not the first choice for immediate volume expansion in children with shock. They are used for replacement of blood loss or correction of some disorders of blood clotting.

Remember to get help if you need to give a crystalloid fluid bolus.

Isotonic Crystalloid Solutions

For a child in shock, the preferred initial fluid for volume replacement is an isotonic crystalloid solution such as

- normal saline
- lactated Ringer's

These fluids are inexpensive and readily available. They also have few complications. To treat hypovolemic shock, you will likely have to give more fluid than the estimated fluid loss.

Rapid infusion of a large volume of fluid is usually well tolerated by a healthy child. A large volume of fluid, however, should not be used in the critically ill child with underlying cardiac or renal disease.

Rate and Volume of Fluid Therapy for Shock

Start fluid therapy for shock with 20 mL/kg of isotonic crystalloid administered as a bolus over 5 to 20 minutes. If you do not know the child's weight, use a length-based tape to quickly estimate it.

Decide the volume of isotonic fluid and rate of delivery based on type of condition:

Type of Condition	Volume of Fluid	Rate of Delivery
• Hypovolemic shock • Distributive shock	20 mL/kg	*Give fluid bolus more rapidly* (ie, over 5 to 10 minutes)[35-37]
• Poor pumping function of the heart	5 to 10 mL/kg (ie, smaller volume of fluid)	*Give fluid bolus more slowly* (ie, over 10 to 20 minutes)

Adjust fluid therapy for conditions such as shock associated with DKA, burns, and some poisonings. See the *PALS Provider Manual* for more information.

Rapid Fluid Delivery

The equipment used for routine pediatric fluid therapy cannot deliver fluid boluses as rapidly as needed for a child in shock. The following are some ways to help deliver fluid more quickly:

- Use a large-diameter catheter, especially if blood or colloid is needed
- Place an inline, 3-way stopcock in the IV tubing system
- Use a 35-mL to 60-mL syringe attached to a 3-way stopcock to push fluids rapidly
- Use a pressure bag (beware of risk of air embolism)
- Consider rapid infusion devices

Note: Use of a rapid infusion rate with an IV infusion pump (eg, entering 999 on an infusion pump) does not provide an adequate fluid delivery rate for children who weigh >20 kg. For example, a 50-kg child with septic shock should ideally receive 1 liter of crystalloid in 15 minutes. It will take 1 hour to deliver this amount of fluid using an infusion pump.

Frequent Reassessment

Frequently reassess the child during fluid resuscitation. Monitor the child to

- assess the response to therapy after each fluid bolus
- determine the need for further fluid boluses
- assess for increased respiratory effort or other signs of fluid in the lungs during and after IV fluid therapy for shock

Watch for these signs that the child's condition is improving:

- decreased respiratory rate (toward normal)
- slowing heart rate (toward normal—not to bradycardia)
- improved peripheral pulses
- improved capillary refill and skin temperature
- improved blood pressure
- increased urinary output
- improved level of consciousness

If the child's clinical condition does not improve, try to identify the cause of shock. This will help you decide the next actions. For example, if capillary refill is still delayed after a fluid bolus, the child may have ongoing bleeding or other fluid loss. If the child's condition gets worse after fluid therapy, suspect cardiogenic or obstructive shock. Increased work of breathing may indicate fluid in the lungs and the need for support of ventilation.

Glucose

Introduction

For a child in shock it is important to monitor blood glucose concentration. Hypoglycemia is a common finding in critically ill children.[38] It can result in brain injury if it is not recognized and effectively treated. Glucose is also necessary for normal heart function, particularly in young infants.

Glucose Monitoring

Measure blood glucose concentration in *all* infants and children with coma, shock, or respiratory failure. Glucose can be measured with a bedside device or central laboratory analysis.

Small infants and chronically ill children have limited stores of glycogen (a substance used to store glucose in the body). These stores may be rapidly depleted during episodes of shock, resulting in hypoglycemia. Infants receiving non–glucose-containing IV fluids are at increased risk for developing hypoglycemia.[39]

> *In all critically ill or injured children, perform a rapid glucose test. This will help rule out hypoglycemia as a cause of shock or a contributing factor to the child's critical condition.*

Diagnosis of Hypoglycemia

Hypoglycemia may be difficult to recognize. Infants and children may have few symptoms even though they are hypoglycemic. Some children may have nonspecific clinical signs of hypoglycemia that may also be signs of other conditions. Nonspecific signs are decreased circulation, tachycardia, hypotension sweating, irritability or lethargy, and hypothermia. These signs may be present with conditions such as low oxygen saturation and shock.

In addition to the measured glucose concentration thresholds listed below, symptomatic hypoglycemia is defined by the presence of clinical signs such as

- decreased circulation
- tachycardia
- sweating
- altered level of consciousness (agitation or lethargy)

Although single values are not applicable to every patient, the following lowest acceptable glucose concentrations can be used to define hypoglycemia[40]:

Age	Consensus Definition of Hypoglycemia
Preterm neonates Term neonates	45 mg/dL or less
Infants Children Adolescents	60 mg/dL or less

The lower range of normal glucose concentration listed in the table is based on samples from fasting infants and children who were not stressed. These numbers may not match the glucose concentration required by a stressed, critically ill, or injured child.

Management of Hypoglycemia

The following are recommendations for managing hypoglycemia:

Decide if ...	Act by giving ...
the glucose concentration is low with minimal symptoms	oral glucose (eg, orange juice or other glucose-containing fluid) as long as the child is not in shock
the glucose concentration is very low or the child is symptomatic	IV/IO dextrose (dextrose is the same as glucose)

Hypoglycemia is treated with IV dextrose (0.5 to 1 g/kg) commonly administered as one of the following:

- $D_{25}W$ (25% dextrose in water) (2 to 4 mL/kg)
- $D_{10}W$ (10% dextrose in water) (5 to 10 mL/kg)

Reassess the blood glucose concentration after administration of dextrose.

Do not infuse dextrose-containing boluses of fluid for treatment of shock. Doing so can cause the child to develop hyperglycemia. This can result in increased urine output and make hypovolemia and shock worse. Electrolyte imbalances can also develop.

> *Remember to get help if you detect a low glucose concentration.*

Part 7

Cardiac Arrest

Introduction	Pediatric cardiac arrest is uncommon. When cardiac arrest does occur, outcome is generally poor. In contrast, outcome from treatment of respiratory failure or shock in children is generally good. The focus therefore should be on prevention of cardiac arrest by

- prevention of disease and injury that can lead to cardiac arrest
- early recognition and management of respiratory distress, respiratory failure, and shock before the condition deteriorates to cardiopulmonary failure and cardiac arrest

> *Detect and treat respiratory failure and shock before the child's condition worsens to cardiopulmonary failure and cardiac arrest.*

This part discusses recognition of cardiopulmonary failure and cardiac arrest using the primary assessment approach. It also discusses the importance of high-quality CPR in management of cardiac arrest.

Learning Objectives

After completing this part you should be able to

- recall that the most common cause of cardiac arrest is progression of respiratory distress and failure or shock, or both
- recognize the clinical signs of cardiopulmonary failure and cardiac arrest
- describe the importance of high-quality CPR in treatment of cardiac arrest
- recall that the heart rhythm in cardiac arrest can be shockable or nonshockable
- state the role of the AED in treatment of cardiac arrest

Types of Cardiac Arrest

The 2 main types of cardiac arrest are

- sudden cardiac arrest
- asphyxial arrest

Sudden cardiac arrest, which is common in adults, is uncommon in children. Sudden cardiac arrest usually results from an acute rhythm disturbance.

Asphyxial arrest is the most common type of cardiac arrest in children. You may have heard the term "asphyxial" used to refer to a condition of choking or suffocation. The term *asphyxial arrest* means that the cardiac arrest is caused by an inadequate supply of oxygen to the tissues. This lack of oxygen can result from the progression of respiratory distress and failure or shock, or both (Figure).

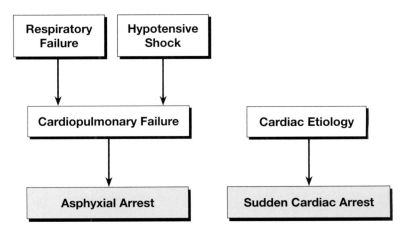

Figure. Pathway to cardiac arrest

Recognition of Cardiopulmonary Failure

You must recognize and treat cardiopulmonary failure quickly. Children in respiratory distress, respiratory failure, or shock develop cardiopulmonary failure immediately before cardiac arrest (Figure 3). Cardiopulmonary failure is the combination of respiratory failure and shock (usually hypotensive). Once the child develops cardiopulmonary failure, the process may be difficult to reverse. You must act quickly to try to prevent cardiac arrest.

Look for the following signs of cardiopulmonary failure during the primary assessment (Table 12).

Table 1. Signs of Cardiopulmonary Failure

Primary Assessment	Signs
A	Possible upper airway obstruction due to decreased level of consciousness
B	• Slow respiratory rate or only agonal gasps • Decreased respiratory effort • Decreased breath sounds
C	• Bradycardia • Absence of peripheral pulses • Weak central pulses • Delayed capillary refill time (typically >5 seconds) • Mottled or cyanotic skin • Cool extremities • Hypotension (usually)
D	Diminished level of consciousness
E	Deferred while addressing life-threatening condition

Recognition of Cardiac Arrest

Clinical Signs of Cardiac Arrest

Cardiac arrest is the loss of blood flow as a result of absent or ineffective heart activity. Signs of circulation are absent. Low levels of oxygen in the brain cause victims to lose consciousness and stop breathing. Agonal gasps may be present in the first minutes after sudden cardiac arrest.

Recognize cardiac arrest by the following clinical signs (Table 13).

Table 2. Clinical Signs of Cardiac Arrest

Primary Assessment	Signs
A	
B	No breathing or only agonal gasps
C	No detectable pulses
D	Unresponsiveness
E	

Because pulse checks may be inaccurate, you can also recognize cardiac arrest by the *absence* of other clinical signs of life, including movement in response to stimulation.

Basic Life Support

Introduction

BLS includes performing high-quality CPR and using an AED. High-quality CPR is the foundation of basic and advanced life support for the management of cardiac arrest. Until the AED arrives, a team member should perform immediate high-quality CPR (Table 14).

Table 14 summarizes the important concepts of BLS.

Table 3. Summary of BLS ABCD Maneuvers for Infants, Children, and Adults

(Newborn/Neonatal Information Not Included) *Note:* Maneuvers used only by healthcare providers are indicated by "HCP."

Maneuver	Adult Lay rescuer: ≥8 years HCP: Adolescent and older	Child Lay rescuers: 1 to 8 years HCP: 1 year to adolescent	Infant Under 1 year of age
ACTIVATE Emergency Response Number (lone rescuer)	Activate when victim found unresponsive **HCP:** if asphyxial arrest likely, call after 5 cycles (2 minutes) of CPR	Activate after performing 5 cycles of CPR For sudden, witnessed collapse, activate after verifying that victim unresponsive	
AIRWAY	Head tilt–chin lift (HCP: suspected trauma, use jaw thrust)		
BREATHS Initial	2 breaths at 1 second/breath	2 effective breaths at 1 second/breath	
HCP: Rescue breathing without chest compressions	10 to 12 breaths/min (approximately 1 breath every 5 to 6 seconds)	12 to 20 breaths/min (approximately 1 breath every 3 to 5 seconds)	
HCP: Rescue breaths for CPR with advanced airway	8 to 10 breaths/min (approximately 1 breath every 6 to 8 seconds)		
Foreign-body airway obstruction	Abdominal thrusts		Back slaps and chest thrusts
CIRCULATION **HCP:** Pulse check (≤10 sec)	Carotid (**HCP** can use femoral in child)		Brachial or femoral
Compression landmarks	Center of chest, between nipples		Just below nipple line
Compression method Push hard and fast Allow complete recoil	**2 Hands:** Heel of 1 hand, other hand on top	**2 Hands:** Heel of 1 hand with second on top or **1 Hand:** Heel of 1 hand only	1 rescuer: 2 fingers **HCP**, 2 rescuers: 2 thumb–encircling hands
Compression depth	1½ to 2 inches	Approximately ⅓ to ½ the depth of the chest	
Compression rate	Approximately 100/min		
Compression- ventilation ratio	30:2 (1 or 2 rescuers)	30:2 (single rescuer) **HCP**: 15:2 (2 rescuers)	
DEFIBRILLATION			
AED	Use adult pads. Do not use child pads/child system. **HCP:** For out-of-hospital response may provide 5 cycles/2 minutes of CPR before shock if response > 4 to 5 minutes and arrest not witnessed.	**HCP:** Use AED as soon as available for sudden collapse and in-hospital. **All:** After about 2 minutes of CPR (out-of-hospital). Use child pads/child system for child 1 to 8 years if available. If child pads/system not available, use adult AED and pads.	No recommendation for infants <1 year of age

High-Quality CPR

To provide high-quality CPR you must perform good chest compressions:

Push hard	• Push with enough force to depress the chest approximately one third to one half the anterior/posterior diameter. • *Release completely,* allowing the chest to fully recoil.
Push fast	Push at a rate of approximately 100 compressions per minute.
Minimize interruptions	• Try to limit interruptions in chest compressions to 10 seconds or less or as needed for interventions (eg, defibrillation). Ideally compressions are interrupted only for ventilation (until an advanced airway is placed), rhythm check, and actual shock delivery. • Once an advanced airway is in place, provide continuous chest compressions.

Remember to push hard, push fast, and minimize interruptions.

Decide Which Actions to Take Based on the Likely Cause of Arrest

Decide which actions to take first based on the likely cause of the arrest.

If the arrest is ...	Then ...
Unwitnessed (assumed to be asphyxial in origin) in the out-of-hospital setting	• Start immediate CPR and send someone to activate the emergency response system and get an AED. • Perform cycles of chest compressions and ventilations for about 2 minutes. • If alone, after about 2 minutes of CPR, activate the emergency response system and get an AED. Return to the victim to give CPR and use the AED.
Witnessed (sudden collapse more likely to be cardiac in origin) and in-hospital arrest	• Send someone to activate the emergency response system and get an AED while you begin CPR. If you are alone, you should activate the emergency response system and get an AED and then begin the steps of CPR. • Use the AED (and follow the voice prompts) as soon as it is available.

Pediatric BLS for Healthcare Providers Algorithm

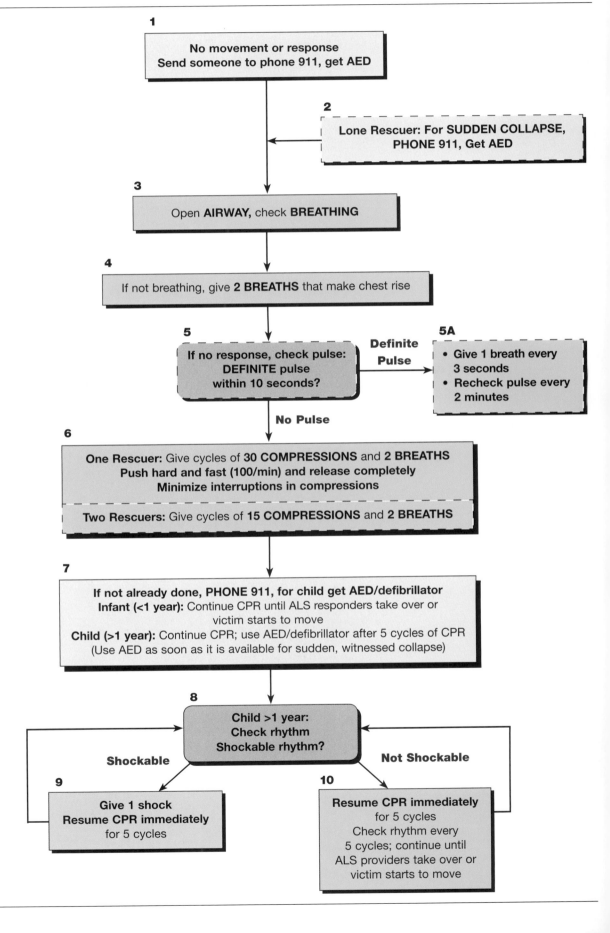

1
No movement or response
Send someone to phone 911, get AED

2
Lone Rescuer: For SUDDEN COLLAPSE,
PHONE 911, Get AED

3
Open **AIRWAY**, check **BREATHING**

4
If not breathing, give **2 BREATHS** that make chest rise

5
If no response, check pulse:
DEFINITE pulse
within 10 seconds?

Definite
Pulse

5A
• Give 1 breath every
3 seconds
• Recheck pulse every
2 minutes

No Pulse

6
One Rescuer: Give cycles of **30 COMPRESSIONS** and **2 BREATHS**
Push hard and fast (100/min) and release completely
Minimize interruptions in compressions

Two Rescuers: Give cycles of **15 COMPRESSIONS** and **2 BREATHS**

7
If not already done, PHONE 911, for child get AED/defibrillator
Infant (<1 year): Continue CPR until ALS responders take over or
victim starts to move
Child (>1 year): Continue CPR; use AED/defibrillator after 5 cycles of CPR
(Use AED as soon as it is available for sudden, witnessed collapse)

8
Child >1 year:
Check rhythm
Shockable rhythm?

Shockable

Not Shockable

9
Give 1 shock
Resume CPR immediately
for 5 cycles

10
Resume CPR immediately
for 5 cycles
Check rhythm every
5 cycles; continue until
ALS providers take over or
victim starts to move

Shockable and Nonshockable Rhythms

The heart rhythms associated with cardiac arrest can be categorized as

- shockable
- nonshockable

Shockable Rhythm

A shockable rhythm is an abnormal rhythm of the heart that can be treated with an electric shock. Shock delivery is also known as defibrillation. A shockable rhythm is the cause of about 5% to 15% of out-of-hospital cardiac arrests in children.[41-43] A shockable rhythm is more likely to be present in a sudden cardiac arrest.

When in-hospital cardiac arrest occurs, a shockable rhythm is initially present in about 10% of arrest victims. At some point in the attempted resuscitation, about 25% of children with cardiac arrest have a shockable rhythm. For this reason it is important to know how to give CPR and use an AED.

Nonshockable Rhythm

A nonshockable rhythm is an abnormal rhythm of the heart that is not treated with defibrillation. Nonshockable rhythms are more common than shockable rhythms in pediatric cardiac arrest. Survival is lower when a cardiac arrest victim presents with a nonshockable rather than a shockable rhythm.[1,44]

Defibrillation

Only shockable rhythms are treated with defibrillation. Defibrillation does not restart the heart. A defibrillation shock "stuns" the heart and allows the natural pacemaker cells of the heart to resume an organized rhythm. The return of an organized rhythm alone, however, does not ensure survival. The organized rhythm must ultimately produce effective pumping of the heart so that blood flow occurs. The return of blood flow is defined by the presence of palpable central pulses.

AED Devices

AED devices are programmed to

- determine if a shockable rhythm is present
- charge to the appropriate dose
- prompt the rescuer to deliver a shock

After the machine is turned on, the AED provides voice and visual prompts to assist the operator. Ideally the AEDs used for children are equipped to deliver a pediatric shock dose.

Manual defibrillators are now manufactured with the capability of operating as AEDs. After the manual defibrillator is turned on in the AED mode, the machine provides voice and visual prompts to assist the operator.

> *When using any AED device, first turn it on. Then follow the AED voice and visual prompts.*

Energy Dose

The energy dose delivered by the AED varies according to guideline recommendations based on weight and age:

Weight/Age	AED Energy Dose
≥25 kg (≥8 years of age)	• Use a standard "adult" AED with adult pad-cable system
<25 kg (≥1 year of age and <8 years of age)	• Use a lower dose if a pediatric system is available • Use an adult system if a pediatric system is not available
<1 year of age	Currently there is insufficient evidence for the AHA to recommend for or against the use of an AED for victims in this age group

Pads

Electrode pads are used to deliver the electrical shock from the AED. Self-adhesive pads reduce the risk of current arcing and can be placed before the arrest. The pads can also be used for monitoring.

Position the pads so that the heart is between them. Place one pad on the upper right side of the chest below the clavicle and the other over the apex of the heart (between the left nipple and the left armpit). Use the largest pads that will fit on the chest wall without touching.[45-47]

 Alternatively place self-adhesive electrode pads in an anterior-posterior position with one just to the left of the sternum and the other over the back. Anterior-posterior placement may be necessary in an infant, particularly if only large electrode pads are available.

Apply firm pressure to create good contact between the pad and the skin.

AED Procedure

Turn the AED on. The AED provides voice and visual prompts to assist the operator.

Immediately after the AED delivers a shock, follow the AED prompts. Resume CPR starting with chest compressions. The AED will direct you to give about 2 minutes of CPR. (For 2 rescuers this will be about 10 cycles of 15 compressions followed by 2 ventilations.)

Every 2 minutes of CPR, the AED will check the rhythm.

If the AED Detects a Shockable Rhythm

If the AED detects a shockable rhythm, it will prompt you to deliver a shock.

Immediately after shock delivery, the AED will direct you to resume CPR, beginning with compressions. If more than 1 rescuer is present, a different rescuer should begin compressions after shock delivery. Continue to follow the AED prompts. Minimize interruptions in chest compressions.

If the AED Detects a Nonshockable Rhythm

If the AED detects a nonshockable rhythm, it will direct you to perform CPR.

If there is any doubt about the presence of a pulse, perform CPR. Chest compressions are unlikely to be harmful to a patient with a spontaneous rhythm but weak pulses.

Part (8)

Resuscitation Team Concept

Effective Team Dynamics

Introduction

Successful teams not only have medical expertise and mastery of resuscitation skills but also demonstrate effective communication and team dynamics. The PEARS Provider Course stresses the importance of team roles and effective team dynamics.

During the course you will have an opportunity to practice different roles of a simulated resuscitation team, including the role of a team leader.

Observe 8 Elements

Look for opportunities during the case simulations to practice and observe the following 8 elements of effective team dynamics. Make notes of examples (positive and negative) that you observe during the course.

Table 2. Effective Team Dynamics Observation Sheet

	Element	Observed
1	Closed-loop communication	
2	Clear messages	
3	Clear roles and responsibilities	
4	Knowing one's limitations	
5	Knowledge sharing	

		Element	Observed
6		Constructive intervention	
7		Reevaluation and summarizing	
8		Mutual respect	

Summary of Team Roles

Roles and Responsibilities

During each case simulation the instructor will take the role of the team leader. Students will rotate through team member roles. The team leader may modify a team member's responsibilities according to his or her scope of practice.

Role	Responsibilities
Team leader (instructor)	In the PEARS Provider Course the instructor is the team leader in all case simulations. The instructor will provide information throughout each case, including findings from the general and primary assessments.
Airway	• Open the airway using manual maneuvers. • Suction with an appropriate device. • Give high-flow or low-flow oxygen at the appropriate rate. • Provide bag-mask ventilation when needed. • Evaluate the child's response to oxygen administration or airway medications. • Rotate with the compressor team member about every 2 minutes during CPR and perform chest compressions consistent with BLS guidelines.
Compressor	• Identify cardiac arrest if present. • Activate the emergency response system. • Initiate chest compressions if needed. • Perform chest compressions consistent with the BLS guidelines for effective compressions. • Rotate the role of compressor with the airway team member about every 2 minutes during CPR. • If CPR is not needed in the case simulation, the compressor should alert the team leader that he is now available to assist elsewhere and then perform the newly assigned role.

Role	Responsibilities
IV/IO Medications	• Use a length-based resuscitation tape. • Ensure IV/IO access. • Give a bolus of isotonic crystalloid. • Evaluate response to fluid bolus. • Obtain blood tests as requested (eg, blood glucose). • Give medications as ordered by the team leader (eg, nebulized albuterol treatment).
Monitor/ defibrillator	• Place the pulse oximeter. • Attach pads/leads. • Operate the monitor/defibrillator or AED. • Safely provide electrical therapy as directed by the AED prompts.
Observer/recorder	This role may be performed by more than 1 student based on the number of students in the station. The instructor will allocate specific responsibilities so that each student is actively involved. • Help the instructor by watching the timer to make sure the simulation lasts no longer than 7 minutes. • Remind compressor and airway team members to rotate about every 2 minutes during CPR. • Locate the appropriate learning station competency checklist in the Appendix to the *PEARS Provider Manual*. • Use this checklist during the case simulation to check off actions performed by each team member. • Listen for examples of positive and negative team dynamics. • Give feedback to team members at the end of the case based on the checklist and observations of team behaviors.

See Figure 4 for location of team members during case simulations.

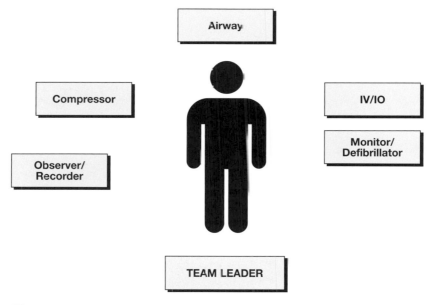

Figure 4. Suggested locations for the team leader and team members during the case simulations.

Appendix

Contents

Introduction

The Appendix contains material that you will use during the course in the skills stations and learning stations. For example, you will use the skills station competency checklists as a guide to skills practice; your instructor will use these checklists to provide feedback. You will use the student CPR practice sheets to prepare for the CPR/AED competency testing lesson. Your instructor will use the CPR Testing Checklist to record your test results.

Course Material

(Continued)

Topic	See page
Learning Station Competency Checklists	
Team Dynamics Practice	
• Cardiac Arrest: Shockable Rhythm	101
• Cardiac Arrest: Nonshockable Rhythm	102
Putting It All Together	
• Upper Airway Obstruction	103
• Lower Airway Obstruction	104
• Lung Tissue Disease	105
• Disordered Control of Breathing	106
• Hypovolemic Shock	107
• Distributive/Septic Shock	108

CPR/AED Practice and Competency Testing

Testing Requirements and Preparation

You must pass 2 CPR tests to receive a course completion card.

Skills Test Requirements
• Pass child 1-rescuer CPR/AED skills test
• Pass infant 1- and 2-rescuer CPR skills test

The PEARS Provider Course does not include detailed instruction on how to do CPR or how to use an AED. You must know this in advance. Consider taking a BLS for Healthcare Providers Course if necessary. Review the student CPR practice sheets, Summary of BLS ABCD Maneuvers (Table 3) and Pediatric BLS Algorithm in Part 7, and CPR testing checklists in this part.

Student CPR Practice Sheets

Introduction

The child 1-rescuer CPR/AED student practice sheet and the infant 1- and 2-rescuer CPR student practice sheet provide detailed descriptions of the CPR skills that you will be expected to perform. Your instructor will evaluate your CPR skills during the skills test based on these descriptions.

If you perform a specific skill exactly as it is described in the critical performance step details, the instructor will check that specific skill as "passing." If you do not perform a specific skill exactly as it is described, the skill will not be checked off, and you will require remediation of that skill.

Study the following student CPR practice sheets so that you will be able to perform each skill correctly.

Child 1-Rescuer CPR/AED Student Practice Sheet

Step	Critical Performance Steps	Details
1	_____ Check for response	Tap victim and ask if the person is "all right" or "OK" speaking loudly and clearly.
2	_____ Activate the emergency response system: Tell someone to phone 911 and get an AED	Activate the emergency response system by making sure that someone phones 911 and gets an AED.
3	_____ Open airway using head tilt–chin lift	Place palm of one hand on forehead and push the head back. Place fingers of other hand under the lower jaw to lift the chin. Do not completely close mouth. Move the head back toward the hand on the forehead in a way that is clearly visible to the instructor.
4	_____ Check for breathing	Place face near the victim's nose and mouth. Look at chest and listen and feel for breathing. Continue for at least 5 seconds but no more than 10 seconds.
5	_____ Give 2 breaths (1 second each) that produce visible chest rise	Use a pocket mask, seal mask around mouth and nose, and give breaths. Give each rescue breath over approximately 1 second. Reposition the head if chest does not rise. You may make multiple attempts to reposition head or improve seal to give breaths that make the chest rise. You should give 2 breaths that produce visible chest rise. Take no more than 10 seconds to accomplish 2 breaths.
6	_____ Check for carotid pulse	Place two or three fingers on the trachea and slip the fingers into the groove between the trachea and muscles on the side of the neck. Check for pulse for at least 5 seconds but no more than 10 seconds.
7	_____ Locate CPR hand position	Move or remove clothing from victim's chest. Place heel of one hand in the center of chest between the nipples. You may place the other hand on top of the first hand (if needed to compress the chest to the correct depth). Extend or interlace fingers to keep off chest.
8	_____ Deliver first cycle of 30 compressions at the correct rate	Keep hand(s) in proper place on chest. Give 30 compressions in less than 23 seconds. Push hard, push fast; allow chest to return to normal between compressions.

Step	Critical Performance Steps	Details
9	_____ Give 2 breaths (1 second each) with visible chest rise	Use a pocket mask, seal mask around mouth and nose, and give breaths.
		Give each rescue breath over approximately 1 second.
		Reposition the head if chest does not rise.
		You may make multiple attempts to reposition head or improve seal to give breaths that make the chest rise.
		You should give 2 breaths that produce visible chest rise.
		Take no more than 10 seconds to accomplish 2 breaths, then move to compressions.
AED Arrives		
AED 1	_____ Turn AED on	Stop CPR and press button to turn AED on (or make sure that AED case is open if your AED has an automatic-on feature).
AED 2	_____ Select proper pads and place pads correctly	You must recognize the difference between adult pads and child pads, select the proper pad size for the child victim, and apply the pads to the chest as illustrated on the pads and/or AED instructions.
AED 3	_____ Clear victim to allow AED to analyze rhythm	Show a visible sign of clearing the victim along with a verbal indication of clearing the victim: "Clear! Stay clear of victim!" or similar statement with an obvious gesture to ensure that all are clear.
AED 4	_____ Clear victim to deliver shock/ Press shock button	Show a visible sign of clearing the victim along with a verbal indication of clearing the victim: "Clear! Stay clear of victim!" or similar statement with an obvious gesture to ensure that all are clear.
		Press shock button when prompted and after clearing.
10	_____ Resume CPR: deliver second cycle of 30 compressions using correct hand position	Resume CPR, beginning with compressions, immediately after shock delivery. Place heel of one hand in the center of chest, between the nipples.
		You may place the other hand on top of the first hand (if needed to compress the chest to the correct depth).
		Extend or interlace fingers to keep off chest.
		Do 30 compressions.
11	_____ Give 2 breaths (1 second each) that produce visible chest rise	Use a pocket mask, seal mask around mouth and nose, and give breaths.
		Give each rescue breath over approximately 1 second.
		Reposition the head if chest does not rise.
		You may make multiple attempts to reposition head or improve seal to give breaths that make the chest rise.
		You should give 2 breaths that produce visible chest rise.
		Take no more than 10 seconds to accomplish 2 breaths and then move to compressions.
12	_____ Deliver third cycle of 30 compressions of adequate depth with chest returning to normal position after each compression	Push hard, push fast; allow chest to return to normal between compressions.
		You must do at least 23 of 30 compressions correctly: adequate depth and allowing the chest to return to normal between compressions.

Infant 1- and 2-Rescuer CPR Student Practice Sheet

Step	Critical Performance Steps	Details
1	_____ Check for response	Tap infant and shout loudly.
2	_____ Activate emergency response system	Tell bystander to activate appropriate emergency response.
3	_____ Open airway using head tilt–chin lift	Push back on manikin forehead; place fingers of other hand on the bony part of the victim's chin, and lift the victim's chin.
		Do not press the soft tissues of the neck or under the chin.
		Lift the jaw upward by bringing the chin forward.
		Do NOT hyperextend the neck.
4	_____ Check for breathing	Place face near the victim's nose and mouth.
		Look at chest and listen and feel for breathing.
		Continue for at least 5 seconds but no more than 10 seconds.
5	_____ Give 2 breaths (1 second each) that produce visible chest rise	Use a pocket mask, seal mask around mouth and nose, and give breaths.
		Give each rescue breath over approximately 1 second.
		Reposition the head if chest does not rise.
		You may make multiple attempts to reposition head or improve seal to give breaths that make the chest rise.
		You should give 2 breaths that produce visible chest rise.
		Take no more than 10 seconds to accomplish 2 breaths.
6	_____ Check for brachial pulse	Locate the brachial pulse in the manikin's upper arm closer to you, using the fingers to try to feel the pulse between the biceps muscle and the humerus.
		Gently feel for a pulse for at least 5 seconds but no more than 10 seconds.
7	_____ Locate CPR finger position	Place 2 fingers on the sternum just below the nipple line.
8	_____ Deliver first cycle of 30 compressions at the correct rate	Give 30 compressions in less than 23 seconds.
		Push hard, push fast; allow chest to return to normal position between compressions.
9	_____ Give 2 breaths (1 second each) that produce visible chest rise	Use a pocket mask, seal mask around mouth and nose, and give breaths.
		Give each rescue breath over approximately 1 second.
		Reposition the head if chest does not rise.
		You should give 2 breaths that produce visible chest rise.
		Take no more than 10 seconds to accomplish 2 breaths, then move to compressions.

Step	Critical Performance Steps	Details
Second rescuer will help perform CPR, taking over rescue breaths, using a bag mask. Rescuers should use a 15:2 compression–to–ventilation ratio.		
10	_____ Deliver cycle of 15 compressions using 2 thumb–encircling hands technique	Compress lower half of sternum with 2 thumb–encircling hands technique in proper position. Squeeze hands while compressing with thumbs. Do 15 compressions.
11	_____ Pause to allow 2nd rescuer to give 2 breaths	Pause compressions to allow 2nd rescuer to give 2 breaths with bag mask.
12	_____ Deliver cycle of 15 compressions of adequate depth with full chest recoil	Push hard, push fast; allow full chest recoil between compressions. Do 15 compressions.
13	_____ Pause to allow 2nd rescuer to give 2 breaths	Pause compressions to allow 2nd rescuer to give 2 breaths with bag mask.
Switch places with little interruption. You take over rescue breaths, using bag mask. Two more CPR cycles are performed.		
14	_____ Give 2 breaths that produce visible chest rise during pauses in compressions using bag mask (2 cycles)	Use bag mask, seal mask properly, and squeeze bag. Two breaths should produce visible chest rise. Breaths should take approximately 1 second each. You may make multiple attempts to reposition head or improve seal to give breaths that make the chest rise. (Sounds of an air leak can be present as long as there is visible chest rise.) Repeat for 2 cycles with 2nd rescuer doing chest compressions.

Remediation

Remediation Lesson   Any student who does not pass both skills tests will practice and be remediated during the Remediation Lesson at the end of the course.

Students who need remediation testing will be tested in the *entire* skill.

PEARS CPR Testing Checklist

Introduction   The instructor will record your skills tests results on the CPR testing checklist:

- The first page of the checklist is for the child CPR + AED skills test.
- The second page is for the infant 1- and 2-rescuer CPR skills test.

Review the CPR testing checklist to understand the criteria your instructor will use to evaluate your skills.

PEARS CPR Testing Checklist

American Heart Association PEARS Child 1-Rescuer CPR and AED Test	Name: _____ Date of Test: _____

Skill Step	Child 1-Rescuer CPR With AED C R I T I C A L P E R F O R M A N C E S T E P S	☑ if done correctly
1	Checks for response	
2	Activates the emergency response system: Tells someone to phone 911 and get an AED	
3	Opens airway using head tilt–chin lift	
4	Checks for breathing *Minimum 5 seconds; maximum 10 seconds*	
5	Gives 2 breaths (1 second each) that produce visible chest rise	
6	Checks for carotid pulse *Minimum 5 seconds; maximum 10 seconds*	
7	Locates CPR hand position	
8	Delivers first cycle of 30 compressions at correct rate *Acceptable <23 seconds for 30 compressions*	
9	Gives 2 breaths (1 second each) that produce visible chest rise	
AED Arrives.		
AED 1	Turns AED On	
AED 2	Selects proper AED pads and places pads correctly	
AED 3	Clears victim to analyze *(Must be visible and verbal check)*	
AED 4	Clears victim to shock/Presses shock button *(Must be visible and verbal check) Maximum time from AED arrival <90 sec*	
Student continues CPR.		
10	Delivers second cycle of 30 compressions at correct hand position *Acceptable >23 of 30 compressions at correct position*	
11	Gives 2 breaths (1 second each) with visible chest rise	
The next step is done only with a manikin with a feedback device, such as a clicker or light. If not, STOP THE TEST.		
12	Delivers third cycle of 30 compressions of adequate depth with full chest recoil *Acceptable >23 comps of 30 with adequate depth and recoil*	

		STOP THE TEST	
		P	NR

CPR TEST RESULTS	Indicate Pass or Needs Remediation	CPR/AED		INFANT	
		P	NR	P	NR
INST SIGNATURE:					

Name: _____

Date of Test: _____

Skill Step	Infant 1- and 2-Rescuer CPR C R I T I C A L P E R F O R M A N C E S T E P S	☑ if done correctly
1	Checks for response	
2	Activates emergency response system	
3	Opens airway using head tilt–chin lift	
4	Checks for breathing *Minimum 5 seconds; maximum 10 seconds*	
5	Gives 2 breaths (1 second each) that produce visible chest rise	
6	Checks for brachial pulse *Minimum 5 seconds; maximum 10 seconds*	
7	Locates CPR finger position	
8	Delivers first cycle of 30 compressions at correct rate *Acceptable <23 seconds for 30 compressions*	
9	Gives 2 breaths (1 second each) with visible chest rise	
Second rescuer arrives and takes over breathing with bag mask. Test only first rescuer. Rescuers use 15:2 ratio.		
10	1st rescuer delivers cycle of 15 compressions using 2 thumb–encircling hands technique *Acceptable >11 of 15 compressions at correct position*	
11	1st rescuer pauses to allow 2nd rescuer to give 2 breaths	
12	1st rescuer delivers cycle of 15 compressions of adequate depth with full chest recoil *Measure depth only if using instrumented manikin; otherwise observe that compressions are given.*	
13	1st rescuer pauses to allow 2nd rescuer to give 2 breaths	
Rescuers switch places with little interruption. 1st rescuer takes over rescue breaths using bag mask. Students perform 2 more cycles of CPR. Test only 1st rescuer.		
14	1st rescuer gives 2 breaths that produce visible chest rise during pauses in compressions using bag mask (2 cycles)	

	STOP THE TEST	
Mark results for this test on bottom of other side	P	NR

Pediatric Assessment

Assess–Categorize–Decide–Act (ACDA)

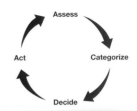

Assess · Categorize · Decide · Act

General Assessment	If at any point during the general assessment you identify a life-threatening problem, immediately start lifesaving actions and get help!

Appearance	**TICLS: T**one, **I**nteractiveness, **C**onsolability, **L**ook/Gaze, **S**peech/Cry		
	All normal?	Any abnormal?	
Work of Breathing	Normal effort	Increased effort Decreased effort	Abnormal sounds
Circulation	Normal skin color, no external bleeding	Abnormal skin color	External bleeding
Not life threatening ➡ *Go to primary assessment*		Life threatening ➡ *Act!*	

Primary Assessment	If at any point during the general assessment you identify a life-threatening problem, immediately start lifesaving actions and get help!

Airway	Clear	Maintainable	Not maintainable

Breathing	Respiratory Rate	Respiratory Effort	Air Movement	Airway and Breath Sounds		Pulse Oximetry
	Normal Fast Slow Apnea	Normal Nasal flaring Chest retractions Head bobbing Seesaw respirations	Normal Decreased	*Airway Sounds* Stridor Barking cough Grunting Gurgling	*Breath Sounds* Prolonged expiration Wheezing Crackles	Normal oxygen saturation Hypoxemia

Circulation	Heart Rate	Pulses		Capillary Refill Time	Skin Color, Temperature	Blood Pressure
	Normal Fast (tachycardia) Slow (bradycardia)	*Peripheral* Normal Weak Absent	*Central* Normal Weak Absent	Normal: 2 seconds or less Delayed: >2 seconds	Pale skin Mottling Cyanosis Warm skin Cool skin	Normal Abnormal

Disability	AVPU Pediatric Response Scale				Pupil Size Reaction to Light		Blood Glucose	
	Alert	Responds to **V**oice	Responds to **P**ain	**U**nresponsive	Normal	Abnormal	Normal	Low

Exposure	Temperature			Skin	
	Normal	High	Low	Rash	Trauma

Assess–Categorize–Decide–Act (ACDA)

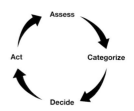

Categorize

Problem	Type	Severity
Respiratory	Upper airway obstruction Lower airway obstruction Lung tissue disease Disordered control of breathing	Respiratory distress Respiratory failure
Circulatory	Hypovolemic shock Distributive shock Cardiogenic shock Obstructive shock	Compensated shock Hypotensive shock
Respiratory + Circulatory	Respiratory type(s) + Circulatory type(s)	Cardiopulmonary failure

Decide

Decide what to do

Act

Begin appropriate actions

Normal Vital Signs

Table 1. Normal Respiratory Rates by Age[3]

Age	Breaths per Minute
Infant (<1 year)	30 to 60
Toddler (1 to 3 years)	24 to 40
Preschooler (4 to 5 years)	22 to 34
School age (6 to 12 years)	18 to 30
Adolescent (13 to 18 years)	12 to 16

Table 3. Oxygen Saturation

Oxygen Saturation Readings	Action
Equal to or greater than 94% when breathing room air	Usually indicates adequate oxygenation; validate by clinical assessment
Less than 94% (hypoxemia) when breathing room air	Consider giving oxygen
Less than 90% in a child receiving 100% oxygen by a nonrebreathing mask (severe hypoxemia)	Call for help; additional actions are usually required

Table 5. Consensus Definition of Hypoglycemia by Age

Age	Consensus Definition of Hypoglycemia
Preterm neonates Term neonates	≤45 mg/dL
Infants Children Adolescents	≤60 mg/dL

Table 2. Normal Heart Rates (per Minute) by Age

Age	Awake Rate	Mean	Sleeping Rate
Newborn to 3 months	85 to 205	140	80 to 160
3 months to 2 years	100 to 190	130	75 to 160
2 years to 10 years	60 to 140	80	60 to 90
>10 years	60 to 100	75	50 to 90

Table 4. Definition of Hypotension by Systolic Blood Pressure and Age

Age	Systolic Blood Pressure (mm Hg)
Term neonates (0 to 28 days)	<60
Infants (1 to 12 months)	<70
Children 1 to 10 years 5th BP percentile	<70 + (age in years × 2)
Children >10 years	<90

Table 6. Normal Blood Pressures in Children by Age

Age	Systolic Blood Pressure (mm Hg)		Diastolic Blood Pressure (mm Hg)	
	Female	Male	Female	Male
Neonate (1st day)	60 to 76	60 to 74	31 to 45	30 to 44
Neonate (4th day)	67 to 83	68 to 84	37 to 53	35 to 53
Infant (1 mo)	73 to 91	74 to 94	36 to 56	37 to 55
Infant (3 mo)	78 to 100	81 to 103	44 to 64	45 to 65
Infant (6 mo)	82 to 102	87 to 105	46 to 66	48 to 68
Infant (1 y)	68 to 104	67 to 103	22 to 60	20 to 58
Child (2 y)	71 to 105	70 to 106	27 to 65	25 to 63
Child (7 y)	79 to 113	79 to 115	39 to 77	38 to 78
Adolescent (15 y)	93 to 127	95 to 131	47 to 85	45 to 85

Respiratory Skills Station
Competency Checklist

Name: _____ **Date of Test:** _____

Critical Performance Steps	☑ if done correctly
Opening the airway	
Opens airway using head tilt–chin lift maneuver while keeping mouth open in the unconscious child (jaw thrust for trauma victim)	
Suctioning	
Demonstrates appropriate use of suction device to remove copious secretions	
Oxygen delivery devices	
Ask student: *"What device delivers a high flow/high concentration of oxygen and what is the correct flow rate?"*	
Verbalizes correct flow rates for the following high-flow/high-concentration device: • Nonrebreathing mask: 10 to 15 L/min	
Ask student: *"What devices deliver a low flow/variable concentration of oxygen and what are the correct flow rates?"*	
Verbalizes correct flow rates for the following low-flow/variable-concentration devices: • Nasal cannula: 0.25 to 4 L/min • Simple oxygen mask: 6 to 10 L/min	
OPA	
Ask student: "When is the OPA used?"	
States that OPA is used only in the unconscious victim without a gag reflex	
Selects correctly sized airway	
Inserts OPA correctly	
Looks, listens, and feels for breathing after insertion of OPA	
Gives 2 breaths (1 second each) with bag mask	
Suctions with OPA in place; states suctioning not to exceed 10 seconds	
Bag-mask device	
Opens airway, uses E-C clamp technique, gives breaths by bag mask, causing observable chest rise. Gives 1 breath every 3 to 5 seconds.	
Respiratory physical exam	
Demonstrates auscultation points for respiratory physical exam	

(Continued)

Optional based on scope of practice: **Nebulizer**	
Identifies components of nebulizer equipment; verbalizes correct oxygen flow settings; verbalizes correct technique for administering medication	
Prepares equipment for delivering medication by nebulizer	
Optional based on scope of practice: **MDI**	
Verbalizes or demonstrates correct technique for administering medication via MDI	

Circulatory Skills Station
Competency Checklist

Name: _____ **Date of Test:** _____

Critical Performance Steps	☑ if done correctly
Monitor/AED	
Applies ECG leads correctly: • White lead: to right shoulder • Red lead: to left ribs, flank • Black, green, or brown lead: to left shoulder	
Demonstrates correct operation of monitor: • Turns monitor on • Checks in lead • Adjusts ECG size and volume • Runs a strip	
Makes correct electrode pad selection for infant or child; places electrode pads in correct position	
Demonstrates safe and correct defibrillation using an AED or manual defibrillator with AED mode	
Vascular access	
Ask student: "What is the next action for a child with poor circulation?"	
Verbalizes that child needs urgent vascular access; calls for help	
Verbalizes that isotonic fluid boluses should be used in shock States appropriate type of fluid to give as a rapid infusion	
Optional based on scope of practice: IV/IO bolus	
Practices giving an IV/IO bolus	
Demonstrates correct use of equipment to give bolus	
Positioning the shock patient	
Demonstrates correct positioning of a child in hypovolemic or distributive shock: lying on the back, face up, with head lowered so that the feet are raised above the level of the heart. (*Note:* This is sometimes called the Trendelenburg position.)	
Epinephrine autoinjector	
Discusses correct technique for administering medication via an epinephrine autoinjector	

Pediatric Assessment Flowchart

General Assessment
Appearance ▲ Work of Breathing ▲ Circulation

Primary Assessment

Airway Breathing Circulation Disability Exposure

Secondary Assessment
(SAMPLE history, focused physical exam, bedside glucose)

Tertiary Assessment
(laboratory studies, x-rays, other tests)

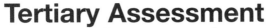

Categorize illness by type and severity

Respiratory	Circulatory
Respiratory distress or *Respiratory failure*	*Compensated shock* or *Hypotensive shock*
Upper airway obstruction Lower airway obstruction Lung tissue disease Disordered control of breathing	Hypovolemic shock Distributive shock Cardiogenic shock Obstructive shock

Respiratory + Circulatory
including cardiopulmonary failure

If at any time during the assessment and categorization process you identify a life-threatening condition

Immediately start life-saving actions

and

activate the emergency response system

Categorize Respiratory Problems by Type

Clinical Signs		Upper Airway Obstruction	Lower Airway Obstruction	Lung Tissue Disease	Disordered Control of Breathing
A	Patency	Airway clear/maintainable/not maintainable			
B	Respiratory Rate/Effort	Increased			Variable
	Air Movement	Decreased			Variable
	Airway and Breath Sounds	Stridor (typically inspiratory) Seal-like cough Hoarseness	Prolonged expiration Wheezing (typically expiratory)	Grunting Crackles Decreased breath sounds	Normal breath sounds Snoring
C	Heart Rate	Tachycardia (early) Bradycardia (late)			
	Skin Color Temperature	Pallor, cool skin (early) Cyanosis (late)			
D	Level of Consciousness	Anxiety, agitation (early) Lethargy, unresponsiveness (late)			
E	Temperature	Variable			

Categorize Respiratory Problems by Severity

	Respiratory Distress ⟶ Respiratory Failure
A	Open and maintainable ⟹ **Not maintainable**
B	Fast respiratory rate ⟹ **Slow respiratory rate to apnea**
	Work of breathing (nasal flaring/retractions) **Increased effort** ⟹ **Decreased effort** ⟹ **Apnea**
	Good air movement ⟹ **Poor to absent air movement**
C	Tachycardia ⟹ **Bradycardia**
	Pallor ⟹ **Cyanosis**
D	Anxiety, agitation ⟹ **Lethargy to unresponsiveness**
E	Variable temperature

Management of Respiratory Emergencies

General Management for All Patients

- Get help *(Note: Give epinephrine first for anaphylaxis)*
- Support airway (positioning, suctioning, manual maneuvers, OPA)
- Assist ventilation if needed
- Give oxygen
- Monitor respiratory rate and effort, oxygen saturation by pulse oximetry, heart rate, level of consciousness
- Ensure vascular access as needed
- Perform frequent reassessments

Upper Airway Obstruction
Specific Management for Selected Conditions

Croup	*Anaphylaxis*	*Other (eg, foreign body, abscess)*
• Nebulized epinephrine	• Epinephrine by autoinjector • Nebulized albuterol (or MDI) PRN • 20 mL/kg NS/LR bolus PRN hypotension	• Remove foreign body if seen • Nebulized epinephrine PRN

Lower Airway Obstruction
Specific Management for Selected Conditions

Bronchiolitis	*Asthma*
• Consider nebulized epinephrine or albuterol	• Nebulized albuterol (or MDI)

Lung Tissue Disease
Specific Management for Selected Conditions

Pneumonia

- Give first dose of antibiotic (after drawing blood cultures)
- Nebulized albuterol (or MDI) PRN
- Treat fever

Disordered Control of Breathing
Specific Management for Selected Conditions

Increased ICP	*Poisoning/Overdose*	*Neuromuscular Disease*
• Elevate head; keep in midline • Treat fever • Assist ventilation (provide hyperventilation if needed)	• Assist ventilation • Contact poison control	• Assist ventilation • Suction as needed

Categorize Shock by Type and Severity

Clinical Signs		Hypovolemic Shock	Distributive/Septic Shock
A	Patency	Airway clear/maintainable/not maintainable	
B	Respiratory rate	Increased	
B	Respiratory effort	Normal to increased	
B	Airway and breath sounds	Normal	Normal (+/− crackles)
C	Heart rate	Increased	
C	Peripheral pulse quality	Weak or absent	Very strong (bounding) or weak
C	Capillary refill time	Delayed	Variable
C	Skin color and temperature	Pale, cool, and/or mottled	Warm or cool
C	Systolic blood pressure	(Normal) **Compensated Shock** ➡	(Below normal) **Hypotensive Shock**
C	Urine output	Decreased	
D	Level of consciousness	Anxiety, agitation (early) Lethargy, unresponsiveness (late)	
E	Temperature	Variable	

Management of Shock

General Management for All Patients
• Get help • Position the child • Give high-flow/high-concentration oxygen • Support ventilation as needed • Ensure vascular (IV/IO) access • Begin IV fluid therapy for shock • Monitor oxygen saturation, heart rate, peripheral pulses, capillary refill, skin color and temperature, blood pressure, urine output, level of consciousness, blood glucose • Perform frequent reassessments
Hypovolemic Shock
• 20 mL/kg NS/LR bolus • Control external bleeding (if present)
Distributive/Septic Shock
• 20 mL/kg NS/LR bolus

Learning Station Competency Checklists

Cardiac Arrest: Shockable Rhythm Team Dynamics Practice	*The observer/recorder should use this checklist during case simulations to check off the performance of team members and provide feedback.*

Critical Performance Steps
Each Team Member
___ Demonstrates effective team dynamics (see "Effective Team Dynamics," below)
Team Member Role: Airway
___ Performs manual maneuvers to open airway*
___ Simulates suctioning of airway*
___ Initiates assisted ventilation with bag-mask device attached to (simulated) high-flow oxygen
___ Simulates administration of high-flow/high-concentration oxygen
___ Performs effective ventilations with bag-mask device
___ Rotates with compressor about every 2 minutes during CPR
Team Member Role: Compressor
___ Begins initial steps of CPR
___ Activates emergency response system
___ Identifies respiratory then cardiac arrest
___ Performs high-quality chest compressions consistent with the BLS Guidelines
___ Rotates compressor role with airway team member about every 2 minutes during CPR
Team Member Role: IV/IO Medications
___ Simulates placement of vascular access (IV/IO)*
Team Member Role: Monitor/Defibrillator
___ Turns on AED
___ Places pads in correct position
___ Follows AED prompts
*If indicated and within student's scope of practice

Effective Team Dynamics	
Closed-loop communication	Knowledge sharing
Clear messages	Constructive intervention
Clear roles and responsibilities	Reevaluation and summarizing
Knowing one's limitations	Mutual respect

Cardiac Arrest: Nonshockable Rhythm Team Dynamics Practice	*The observer/recorder should use this checklist during case simulations to check off the performance of team members and provide feedback.*

Critical Performance Steps

Each Team Member

___ Demonstrates effective team dynamics (see "Effective Team Dynamics," below)

Team Member Role: Airway

___ Performs manual maneuvers to open airway*

___ Simulates suctioning of airway*

___ Initiates assisted ventilation with bag-mask device attached to (simulated) high-flow oxygen*

___ Performs effective ventilations with bag-mask device*

___ Rotates with compressor about every 2 minutes during CPR

Team Member Role: Compressor

___ Begins initial steps of CPR

___ Activates emergency response system

___ Identifies respiratory then cardiac arrest

___ Performs high-quality chest compressions consistent with the BLS guidelines

___ Rotates role of compressor with airway team member about every 2 minutes during CPR

Team Member Role: IV/IO Medications

___ Simulates placement of vascular access (IV/IO)*

___ Simulates administration of medications as directed

Team Member Role: Monitor/Defibrillator

___ Turns on AED

___ Places pads in correct position

___ Follows AED prompts

If indicated and within student's scope of practice

Effective Team Dynamics

Closed-loop communication	**Knowledge sharing**
Clear messages	**Constructive intervention**
Clear roles and responsibilities	**Reevaluation and summarizing**
Knowing one's limitations	**Mutual respect**

Upper Airway Obstruction Putting It All Together	The observer/recorder should use this checklist during case simulations to check off the performance of team members and provide feedback.

Critical Performance Steps

Each Team Member

___ Demonstrates effective team dynamics (see "Effective Team Dynamics," below)

Team Member Role: Airway

___ Recognizes signs and symptoms of a respiratory problem

___ Opens airway*

___ Simulates suctioning of airway*

___ Simulates administration of supplementary oxygen with appropriate delivery device

___ Categorizes severity of respiratory problem

___ Categorizes type of respiratory problem

___ Evaluates response to administration of supplementary oxygen and airway medication

Team Member Role: Compressor

___ Activates emergency response system

___ Assists other team members as directed by team leader

Team Member Role: IV/IO Meds

___ Simulates administration of nebulized epinephrine treatment*

Team Member Role: Monitor/Defibrillator

___ Simulates placement of pulse oximeter

___ Places ECG leads in correct position

___ Turns on monitor

If indicated and within student's scope of practice

Effective Team Dynamics

Closed-loop communication

Clear messages

Clear roles and responsibilities

Knowing one's limitations

Knowledge sharing

Constructive intervention

Reevaluation and summarizing

Mutual respect

Lower Airway Obstruction **Putting It All Together**	The observer/recorder should use this checklist during case simulations to check off the performance of team members and provide feedback.

Critical Performance Steps

Each Team Member

___ Demonstrates effective team dynamics (see "Effective Team Dynamics," below)

Team Member Role: Airway

___ Recognizes signs and symptoms of a respiratory problem

___ Opens airway*

___ Simulates suctioning of airway*

___ Simulates administration of supplementary oxygen with appropriate delivery device

___ Categorizes severity of respiratory problem

___ Categorizes type of respiratory problem

___ Evaluates response to administration of supplementary oxygen and airway medication

Team Member Role: Compressor

___ Activates emergency response system

___ Assists other team members as directed by team leader

Team Member Role: IV/IO Medications

___ Simulates administration of nebulized albuterol treatment*

Team Member Role: Monitor/Defibrillator

___ Simulates placement of pulse oximeter

___ Places ECG leads in correct position

___ Turns on monitor

If indicated and within student's scope of practice

Effective Team Dynamics

Closed-loop communication	Knowledge sharing
Clear messages	Constructive intervention
Clear roles and responsibilities	Reevaluation and summarizing
Knowing one's limitations	Mutual respect

Lung Tissue Disease **Putting It All Together**	*The observer/recorder should use this checklist during case simulations to check off the performance of team members and provide feedback.*

Critical Performance Steps

Each Team Member

___ Demonstrates effective team dynamics (see "Effective Team Dynamics," below)

Team Member Role: Airway

___ Recognizes signs and symptoms of a respiratory problem

___ Opens airway*

___ Simulates suctioning of airway*

___ Simulates administration of supplementary oxygen with appropriate delivery device

___ Categorizes severity of respiratory problem

___ Categorizes type of respiratory problem

___ Evaluates response to administration of supplementary oxygen

___ Initiates assisted ventilation with bag-mask device attached to high-flow oxygen*

Team Member Role: Compressor

___ Activates emergency response system

___ Assists other team members as directed by team leader

Team Member Role: IV/IO Medications

___ Simulates placement of vascular access (IV/IO)*

___ Simulates obtaining blood cultures*

___ Simulates administration of medications (ie, antibiotics, antipyretics)

Team Member Role: Monitor/Defibrillator

___ Simulates placement of pulse oximeter

___ Places ECG leads in correct position

___ Turns on monitor

*If indicated and within student's scope of practice

Effective Team Dynamics

Closed-loop communication	**Knowledge sharing**
Clear messages	**Constructive intervention**
Clear roles and responsibilities	**Reevaluation and summarizing**
Knowing one's limitations	**Mutual respect**

Disordered Control of Breathing Putting It All Together	*The observer/recorder should use this checklist during case simulations to check off the performance of team members and provide feedback.*

Critical Performance Steps

Each Team Member

___ Demonstrates effective team dynamics (see "Effective Team Dynamics," below)

Team Member Role: Airway

___ Recognizes signs and symptoms of a respiratory problem

___ Opens airway*

___ Simulates suctioning of airway*

___ Simulates insertion of oropharyngeal airway*

___ Initiates assisted ventilation with bag-mask device attached to (simulated) high-flow oxygen*

___ Categorizes severity of respiratory problem

___ Categorizes type of respiratory problem

___ Evaluates response to assisted ventilation

Team Member Role: Compressor

___ Activates emergency response system

___ Assists other team members as directed by team leader

Team Member Role: IV/IO Medications

___ Simulated placement of vascular access (IV/IO)*

___ Assists other team members as directed by team leader

Team Member Role: Monitor/Defibrillator

___ Simulates placement of pulse oximeter

___ Places ECG leads in correct position

___ Turns on monitor

If indicated and within student's scope of practice

Effective Team Dynamics

Closed-loop communication	Knowledge sharing
Clear messages	Constructive intervention
Clear roles and responsibilities	Reevaluation and summarizing
Knowing one's limitations	Mutual respect

Hypovolemic Shock **Putting It All Together**	*The observer/recorder should use this checklist during case simulations to check off the performance of team members and provide feedback.*

Critical Performance Steps

Each Team Member

___ Demonstrates effective team dynamics (see "Effective Team Dynamics," below)

Team Member Role: Airway

___ Recognizes signs and symptoms of respiratory distress

___ Opens airway*

___ Simulated suctioning of airway*

___ Simulates administration of supplementary oxygen with appropriate delivery device*

___ Evaluates response to administration of supplementary oxygen

Team Member Role: Compressor

___ Activates emergency response system

___ Assists other team members as directed by team leader

Team Member Role: IV/IO Meds

___ Recognizes signs and symptoms of a circulatory problem

___ Categorizes severity of shock

___ Categorizes type of shock

___ Simulates use of length-based resuscitation tape

___ Simulates placement of vascular access (IV/IO)*

___ Simulates administration of 20 mL/kg isotonic crystalloid bolus IV

___ Simulates obtaining rapid glucose test

___ Evaluates response to fluid bolus

Team Member Role: Monitor/Defibrillator

___ Simulates placement of pulse oximeter

___ Places ECG leads in correct position

___ Turns on monitor

*If indicated and within student's scope of practice

Effective Team Dynamics

Closed-loop communication	**Knowledge sharing**
Clear messages	**Constructive intervention**
Clear roles and responsibilities	**Reevaluation and summarizing**
Knowing one's limitations	**Mutual respect**

Distributive/Septic Shock Putting It All Together	The observer/recorder should use this checklist during case simulations to check off the performance of team members and provide feedback.

Critical Performance Steps

Each Team Member

___ Demonstrates effective team dynamics (see "Effective Team Dynamics," below)

Team Member Role: Airway

___ Recognizes signs and symptoms of respiratory distress

___ Opens airway*

___ Simulates suctioning of airway*

___ Simulates administration of supplementary oxygen with appropriate delivery device*

Team Member Role: Compressor

___ Activates emergency response system

___ Assists other team members as directed by team leader

Team Member Role: IV/IO Medications

___ Recognizes signs and symptoms of a circulatory problem

___ Categorizes severity of shock

___ Categorizes type of shock

___ Simulates use of length-based resuscitation tape

___ Simulates placement of vascular access (IV/IO)*

___ Simulates administration of 20 mL/kg isotonic crystalloid bolus IV/IO*

___ Simulates obtaining rapid glucose test and blood cultures*

___ Evaluates response to fluid bolus

___ Simulates administration of medications (ie, antibiotics, antipyretics)*

Team Member Role: Monitor/Defibrillator

___ Simulates placement of pulse oximeter

___ Places ECG leads in correct position

___ Turns on monitor

If indicated and within student's scope of practice

Effective Team Dynamics

Closed-loop communication	**Knowledge sharing**
Clear messages	**Constructive intervention**
Clear roles and responsibilities	**Reevaluation and summarizing**
Knowing one's limitations	**Mutual respect**

References

1. Nadkarni VM, Larkin GL, Peberdy MA, et al. First documented rhythm and clinical outcome from in-hospital cardiac arrest among children and adults. *JAMA.* 2006;295:50-57.

2. Dieckmann R, ed. *Pediatric Education for Prehospital Professionals.* Sudbury, Mass: Jones and Bartlett Publishers, American Academy of Pediatrics; 2006.

3. Hazinski M. Children are different. In: Hazinski M, ed. *Manual of Pediatric Critical Care.* St. Louis, Mo: Mosby-Year Book; 1999.

4. Singer JI, Losek JD. Grunting respirations: chest or abdominal pathology? *Pediatr Emerg Care.* 1992;8:354-358.

5. Gillette PC, Garson A Jr, Porter CJ, et al. Dysrhythmias. In: Adams FH, Emmanouildies GC, Riemenschneider TA, eds. *Moss' Heart Disease in Infants, Children and Adolescents.* 4th ed. Baltimore, MD: Williams & Wilkins; 1989:725-741.

6. Gorelick MH, Shaw KN, Baker MD. Effect of ambient temperature on capillary refill in healthy children. *Pediatrics.* 1993;92:699-702.

7. National High Blood Pressure Education Program Working Group on High Blood Pressure in Children and Adolescents. The fourth report on the diagnosis, evaluation, and treatment of high blood pressure in children and adolescents. *Pediatrics* 2004;114(Suppl):1-22.

8. Gemelli M, Manganaro R, Mami C, et al. Longitudinal study of blood pressure during the 1st year of life. *Eur J Pediatr.* 1990;149:318-320.

9. *Fourth report on the Diagnosis, Evaluation, and Treatment of High Blood Pressure in Children and Adolescents:* NHLBI; May 2004.

10. Hannan EL, Farrell LS, Meaker PS, et al. Predicting inpatient mortality for pediatric trauma patients with blunt injuries: a better alternative. *J Pediatr Surg.* 2000;35:155-159.

11. Skrifvars MB, Saarinen K, Ikola K, et al. Improved survival after in-hospital cardiac arrest outside critical care areas. *Acta Anaesthesiol Scand.* 2005;49:1534-1539.

12. Geelhoed GC, Turner J, Macdonald WB. Efficacy of a small single dose of oral dexamethasone for outpatient croup: a double blind placebo controlled clinical trial. *BMJ.* 1996;313:140-142.

13. Westley CR, Cotton EK, Brooks JG. Nebulized racemic epinephrine by IPPB for the treatment of croup: a double-blind study. *Am J Dis Child.* 1978;132:484-487.

14. Kristjansson S, Berg-Kelly K, Winso E. Inhalation of racemic adrenaline in the treatment of mild and moderately severe croup. Clinical symptom score and oxygen saturation measurements for evaluation of treatment effects. *Acta Paediatr.* 1994;83:1156-1160.

15. Taussig LM, Castro O, Beaudry PH, et al. Treatment of laryngotracheobronchitis (croup). Use of intermittent positive-pressure breathing and racemic epinephrine. *Am J Dis Child.* 1975;129:790-793.

16. Luria JW, Gonzalez-del-Rey JA, DiGiulio GA, et al. Effectiveness of oral or nebulized dexamethasone for children with mild croup. *Arch Pediatr Adolesc Med.* 2001;155:1340-1345.

17. Kairys SW, Olmstead EM, O'Connor GT. Steroid treatment of laryngotracheitis: a meta-analysis of the evidence from randomized trials. *Pediatrics.* 1989;83:683-693.

18. Gold MS, Sainsbury R. First aid anaphylaxis management in children who were prescribed an epinephrine autoinjector device (EpiPen). *J Allergy Clin Immunol.* 2000;106(Pt 1):171-176.

19. Dibs SD, Baker MD. Anaphylaxis in children: a 5-year experience. *Pediatrics.* 1997;99:E7.

20. Sampson HA, Mendelson L, Rosen JP. Fatal and near-fatal anaphylactic reactions to food in children and adolescents. *N Engl J Med.* 1992;327:380-384.

21. Ralston S, Hartenberger C, Anaya T, et al. Randomized, placebo-controlled trial of albuterol and epinephrine at equipotent beta-2 agonist doses in acute bronchiolitis. *Pediatr Pulmonol.* 2005;40:292-299.

22. Patel H, Platt R, Lozano JM, et al. Glucocorticoids for acute viral bronchiolitis in infants and young children. *Cochrane Database Syst Rev.* 2004:CD004878.

23. Schuh S, Coates AL, Binnie R, et al. Efficacy of oral dexamethasone in outpatients with acute bronchiolitis. *J Pediatr.* 2002;140:27-32.

24. Langley JM, Smith MB, LeBlanc JC, et al. Racemic epinephrine compared to salbutamol in hospitalized young children with bronchiolitis; a randomized controlled clinical trial. *BMC Pediatr.* 2005;5:7.

25. Ray MS, Singh V. Comparison of nebulized adrenaline versus salbutamol in wheeze associated respiratory tract infection in infants. *Indian Pediatr.* 2002;39:12-22.

26. Bertrand P, Aranibar H, Castro E, et al. Efficacy of nebulized epinephrine versus salbutamol in hospitalized infants with bronchiolitis. *Pediatr Pulmonol.* 2001;31:284-288.

27. Ciarallo L, Sauer AH, Shannon MW. Intravenous magnesium therapy for moderate to severe pediatric asthma: results of a randomized, placebo-controlled trial. *J Pediatr.* 1996;129:809-814.

28. Khine H, Fuchs SM, Saville AL. Continuous vs intermittent nebulized albuterol for emergency management of asthma. *Acad Emerg Med.* 1996;3:1019-1024.

29. Stephanopoulos DE, Monge R, Schell KH, et al. Continuous intravenous terbutaline for pediatric status asthmaticus. *Crit Care Med.* 1998;26:1744-1748.

30. Ciarallo L, Brousseau D, Reinert S. Higher-dose intravenous magnesium therapy for children with moderate to severe acute asthma. *Arch Pediatr Adolesc Med.* 2000;154:979-983.

31. Plotnick LH, Ducharme FM. Combined inhaled anticholinergic agents and beta-2-agonists for initial treatment of acute asthma in children. *Cochrane Database Syst Rev.* 2000:CD000060.

32. Smith M, Iqbal S, Elliott TM, et al. Corticosteroids for hospitalised children with acute asthma. *Cochrane Database Syst Rev.* 2003:CD002886.

33. Michelow IC, Olsen K, Lozano J, et al. Epidemiology and clinical characteristics of community-acquired pneumonia in hospitalized children. *Pediatrics.* 2004;113:701-707.

34. Carcillo JA. Pediatric septic shock and multiple organ failure. *Crit Care Clin.* 2003;19:413-440, viii.

35. Powell KR, Sugarman LI, Eskenazi AE, et al. Normalization of plasma arginine vasopressin concentrations when children with meningitis are given maintenance plus replacement fluid therapy. *J Pediatr.* 1990;117:515-522.

36. Carcillo JA, Davis AL, Zaritsky A. Role of early fluid resuscitation in pediatric septic shock. *JAMA.* 1991;266:1242-1245.

37. Ceneviva G, Paschall JA, Maffei F, et al. Hemodynamic support in fluid-refractory pediatric septic shock. *Pediatrics.* 1998;102:e19.

38. Losek JD. Hypoglycemia and the ABC'S (sugar) of pediatric resuscitation. *Ann Emerg Med.* 2000;35:43-46.

39. Parker MM, Hazelzet JA, Carcillo JA. Pediatric considerations. *Crit Care Med.* 2004;32(Suppl):S591-594.

40. Cornblath M, Hawdon JM, Williams AF, et al. Controversies regarding definition of neonatal hypoglycemia: suggested operational thresholds. *Pediatrics.* 2000;105:1141-1145.

41. Appleton GO, Cummins RO, Larson MP, et al. CPR and the single rescuer: at what age should you "call first" rather than "call fast"? *Ann Emerg Med.* 1995;25:492-494.

42. Hickey RW, Cohen DM, Strausbaugh S, et al. Pediatric patients requiring CPR in the prehospital setting. *Ann Emerg Med.* 1995;25:495-501.

43. Mogayzel C, Quan L, Graves JR, et al. Out-of-hospital ventricular fibrillation in children and adolescents: causes and outcomes. *Ann Emerg Med.* 1995;25:484-491.

44. Young KD, Gausche-Hill M, McClung CD, et al. A prospective, population-based study of the epidemiology and outcome of out-of-hospital pediatric cardiopulmonary arrest. *Pediatrics.* 2004;114:157-164.

45. Atkins DL, Sirna S, Kieso R, et al. Pediatric defibrillation: importance of paddle size in determining transthoracic impedance. *Pediatrics.* 1988;82:914-918.

46. Atkins DL, Kerber RE. Pediatric defibrillation: current flow is improved by using "adult" electrode paddles. *Pediatrics.* 1994;94:90-93.

47. Samson RA, Atkins DL, Kerber RE. Optimal size of self-adhesive preapplied electrode pads in pediatric defibrillation. *Am J Cardiol.* 1995;75:544-545.

Index